Haṭha Yoga Pradīpikā

Translation with

Notes from Krishnamacharya

TRANSLATED BY

A. G. MOHAN

&

DR. GANESH MOHAN

ISBN-13: 978-981-11-3133-2

Publisher: Svastha Yoga

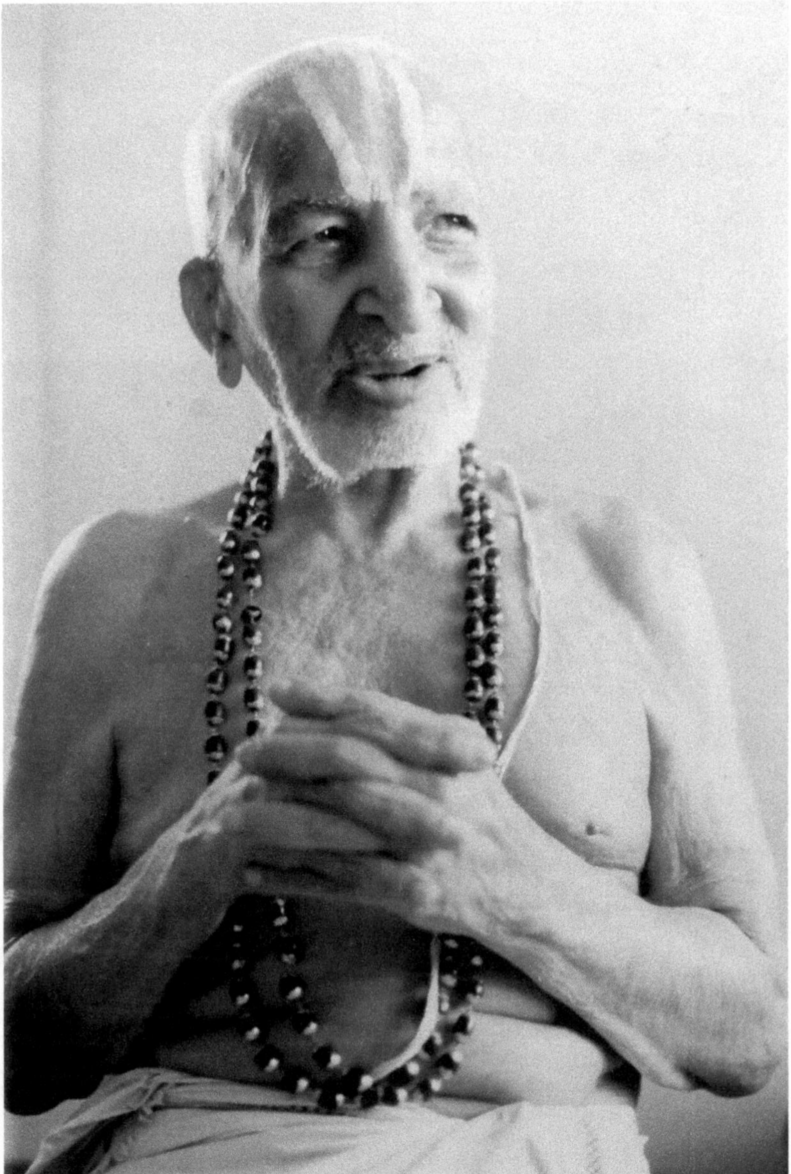

At 100 years

This book is dedicated to

Sāṁkhya-yoga-śikhāmaṇi, Mīmāṁsa-ratna, Mīmāṁsa-tīrtha, Nyāyācārya, Vedānta-vagīśa, Veda-kesari, Yogācārya Sri T. Krishnamacharya.

Haṭha-Yoga in Practice: A. G. Mohan

1973	2017
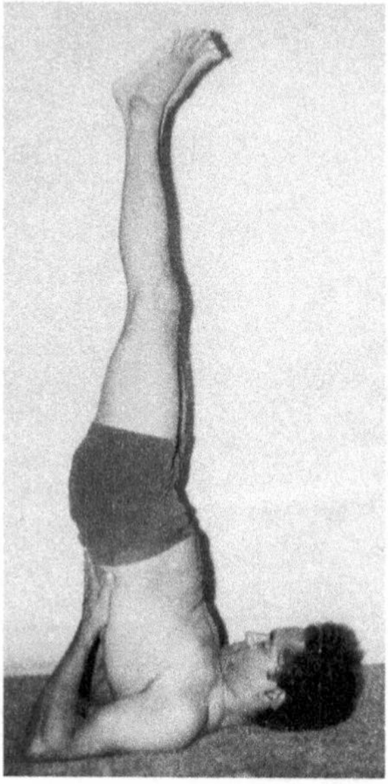	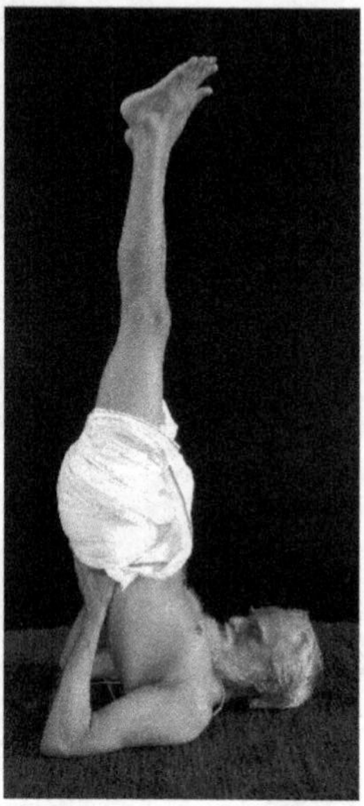
Age: 27 years	Age: 71 years
Under the tutelage of Krishnamacharya	44 years later

Contents

Introduction

Haṭha Yoga Pradīpikā as a Text

As traditional texts on yoga go, the Yoga Sūtra of Patañjali with the commentary of Vyāsa and sub-commentaries is a masterpiece filled with insight. It is clear: all the terms used are clearly defined. It is consistent: it does not contradict itself. It makes a robust effort to be complete: it tries to address all the concepts you need to know to understand the subject. The Yoga Sūtra is the only yoga text that truly offers profound insights for positive self-growth upon repeated reading, reflection, and practice.

The Yoga Yājñavalkya comes reasonably close to being clear and consistent, and somewhat complete.

Now coming to the present work, while is customary for the translator to laud the value of the text being translated, the Haṭha Yoga Pradīpikā already has a somewhat disproportionately high reputation in modern yoga. We prefer to take an objective view, in the best interest of the reader.

Objectively, the Haṭha Yoga Pradīpikā (like other yoga texts except for the Yoga Sūtra and Yoga Yājñavalkya) suffers from being unclear, inconsistent, and incomplete.

Among its flaws: One, it exaggerates and wildly praises the practices it suggests (sphīta-doṣa). Two, it repeats itself unnecessarily in many places (punarukti-doṣa), using several verses where fewer will do, especially in sections of such praise. Three, it does not exercise much discrimination in selecting or evaluating the practices it suggests; some of the practices are simply not very useful or are harmful. (e.g. look at IV.35 and 36—the verses contradict each other.)

The main commentary on the text by Brahmānanda has some interesting points to make, but overall, they amount to perhaps a dozen useful pieces. We have included those pieces of insight or information in the notes under the verses.

To practice or understand what can be practiced or understood from this text, safely and effectively, you need information, insight, and guidance that is not found anywhere in this text itself or its commentary. To understand haṭha-yoga, in-depth study of the Yoga Sūtra and Sāṁkhya is indispensable, familiarity with some of the other tantra texts is important, and some modern neurobiology is very helpful.

So, the Haṭha Yoga Pradīpikā is not a text to be studied with great reverence to detail or meticulously in depth.

Yet, for all its flaws, it is an important text on haṭha-yoga, and does contain valuable insights and practices. To extract that insight, an expert presentation on the Haṭha Yoga Pradīpikā should analyze it with a discriminating eye, discarding the portions that are repetitive, exaggerated, and sometimes just harmful or irrelevant. The presentation should summarize and annotate the key points, and preferably provide comparison to a sister text (the closest ones are likely the Gheraṇḍa Samhitā and Yoga Yājñavalkya) for context in relevant places. It is also important to provide alternatives to some of the less effective and potentially harmful practices in this text. Krishnamacharya followed precisely this approach when teaching this text.

That is what we offer in this book.

What is Yoga?

To answer this, we must look to the foundational work on yoga, the Yoga Sūtra of Patañjali.

In a nutshell, yoga is *sāttvika-samādhi.* That is, yoga is to be stable in a clear, pleasant, and calm life experience. Such a state of mind and body is called *sattva* in Sanskrit. In the body, this state is experienced as vitality and wellness, without restlessness or dullness. In the mind, this is experienced as calmness, with clarity and energy. Generally, this is what all of us want in our lives.

This state of well-being and balance in body and mind is also compositely called *svastha* in yoga and ayurveda.

Patañjali's yoga framework is exceptionally clear, consistent, and complete. It organizes body-mind practices based on ethics, emotions, thoughts, body sensations and movements, breath sensations and movements, sensory changes, visualizations, meditation, and mindfulness.

All other yoga pathways fit within this framework. Logically, they should, because of the wide and comprehensive coverage of Patañjali's eight limbs of yoga.

The key to the state of *svastha* in Patañjali's yoga is yogic mindfulness or meditation, called *smṛti-sādhana*, literally, the "practice of recall." That is, we repeatedly recall our awareness to a calm, clear experience (which could be grounded in breathing, mantra, compassion or one of many other valid meditation possibilities).

There is no progress in yoga without this practice of meditation or yogic mindfulness or recalling one's awareness to a state of *sattva.*

As we repeat this practice, over weeks, months, and years, the mind and body become habitually sattva dominant—calm, clear, pleasant, and stable much of the time. The experience of sattva that we have worked on consciously gradually becomes effortless and natural over time. Then our life experience from day to day and minute to minute is transformed positively.

What is Haṭha-Yoga?

This question requires a deeper answer than we have space to present in this introduction (we expect to give it due attention in a separate work). We will present a summary here.

The ultimate goal of classical haṭha-yoga is the same as that of the Yoga Sūtra, to lead to an experience of sattva (calm, clear, pleasant, stable, light) state of mind and body—a state of svastha.

On what is that experience of sattva or state of svastha based? In haṭha-yoga, that experience is based on the inner awareness of the body. The haṭha-yogi chooses to meditate on, or deepen awareness of, the subtler sensations and experiences in the body, and work with the mind-body connection as a basis of self-transformation.

The practices such as āsana, prāṇāyāma, bandha-s, and mudrā-s, and the terms such as prāṇa, nāḍī, cakra, and kuṇḍalinī are all based on this central concept. They are all practices or descriptions centered on inner body sensations and the mind-body connection. To understand any of these practices or descriptions, it is essential to be clear on this.

The word "prāṇa" is key to descriptions of practices in haṭha-yoga. Prāṇa is often explained to be "life force," which is an accurate translation in some contexts; but it is also an esoteric and not particularly illuminating translation, and not always accurate as the word prāṇa does not always refer to life force *per se*.

The continuous activity of body functions and deep or subtle body sensations are collated under the word prāṇa. When the yogi brings awareness to the subtle inner body sensations, he is "feeling the prana." When awareness is brought to the body like this, the activities or functions happening there will also change. This can in turn change the sensations too. Thus the "flow" or "experience" of "prāṇa" can be altered. Changes in food habits and sensory inputs also play an important role.

Prāṇa as "life force," or the essence of countless ongoing processes that keep organisms alive, does not exist as an entity in our perception. It is intangible and outside our awareness; it is life activity that keeps awareness going at all. What exists in our perception is subtle body sensation. This sensation can have many layers. The more stable and refined your awareness, the more subtle the body sensations you can experience.

But the mind and body are not separate from each other (we have only one nervous system, one hormonal system and so on, from which the functions of the mind also arise, physically). So, focusing on parts of the body, particularly some neurologically significant centers, can be associated with sensations and emotions arising or changing, and can affect the process of self-transformation.

One aspect of haṭha-yoga is using these practices to change the sensations and functions of the body, for preventative or therapeutic goals—to maintain or restore health. That, however, is not the principal focus of the practices in classical haṭha-yoga texts.

The principal focus in classical haṭha-yoga texts is a different aspect: using these practices to work toward changing the sense of self, and going into deeper meditation.

How does this work? The yogi withdraws all the sensations of subtler body awareness deeper into the body, into the spinal cord (or heart center). This is called the "prāṇa being in the suṣumnā." Body functions slow down and sensations diminish. This leads to glimpses of the experience, "I am not my body," and forms the platform for further meditation.

From this point, this text speaks of the practice of "nādānusandhāna," which is meditating on even more subtle sensations in the body, and feels like a sound or vibration. This will eventually lead to a sattva-dominant, stable experience of the root of body sensation and the mind-body connection, an expanded state of awareness, and establish the yogi stably in the feeling, "I am not my body."

Here, the pathway merges into the rest of the Yoga Sūtra. Because the yogi feels that he has an existence beyond the body, he loses fear of death, a point mentioned several times in this text.

Āsana, Prāṇāyāma, Mudrā-s

Let us look at the important features of the steps in the above pathway.

The foundation in haṭha-yoga is āsana. Good health and reasonable comfort are important for the body to be a platform for stable and clear awareness during meditation. This part is not unique to haṭha-yoga; it is the same in the Yoga Sūtra.

In haṭha-yoga, āsana serves as a pathway to general health, and a good mind-body connection, but it is also crucial in awakening subtler sensations in the body. When an āsana (body position with deep and controlled breathing) is used to help feel deeper sensations in the body, it is called a mudrā. For example, the seated forward fold (paścimatānāsana) can be used to feel the sensations in the root (mūla) of the body, if done with deep exhalation, staying for several breaths. The practice of bandha-s in āsana is done with this in mind—hence the bandha-s are a type of mudrā.

A mudrā is a practice that constrains or channels the subtle sensation and activity (prāṇa) in the body, which in turn facilitates stabilizing one's awareness on that sensation. When mūla-bandha (which is based, in simple terms, on pelvic floor engagement and sensation) is practiced, the sensations and activity in that pelvic floor region transition from being open ended and unconstrained to more constrained or channeled. For instance, gently activating the pelvic floor and noticing it constrains the range of sensations and activities that were present there earlier and channels it into a more limited range.

The key here, however, is that the constraint should result in an experience of sattva. That is, it should not feel as if the pelvic floor is under tension or strain, or that the experience of mūla-bandha is unpleasant. That will be rajas (excessively active) or tamas (dull or unclear). Instead, the feeling generated by engaging the pelvic floor region with awareness, when practicing mūla bandha, should be pleasant and comfortable.

Once the yogi feels this inner sensation through mudrā, he repeatedly practices this in appropriate āsana-s, and makes the experience consistent, steadier, and subtler.

Then the yogi incorporates the feeling of the mudrā into prāṇāyāma practice. By controlling the breathing, doing prāṇāyāma with mudrā-s or bandha-s, the yogi can focus awareness on subtle deep body sensations better. When the breath is paused, the activities in the body reduce further, enhancing awareness of inner body sensation. Combining the stopping of the breath with the meditation on the inner awareness of the mudrā-s, the yogi's progress toward absorption in subtle body sensation accelerates.

This lays the platform for further practices of meditation including nādānusandhāna (feeling the subtlest vibrations or sensations in the body).

This is the pathway of classical haṭha-yoga.

Haṭha-Yoga and History

Our expertise and interest is in elucidating the understanding and applications of yoga as a mind-body well-being and self-transformation system, rather than historical, sociological, or political factors in its evolution.

To give an analogy from medicine, knowing the history of how medical science and techniques evolved is of modest use at the time of treating a patient and making clinical decisions on their health. But knowing physiology, pathology, and treatment is crucial and directly relevant.

Similarly, we can understand haṭha-yoga usefully, both theory and practice, only by comprehending *what effect* they have on body and mind, and *who* they are for. The history that led to a practice evolving in a certain form may be interesting, but that by itself says not too much about the use and effectiveness of a practice.

That said, it is certain that haṭha-yoga practices in their essential form have been around for many centuries.

Tantric Sex Practices, Kāpālika-s

The Haṭha Yoga Pradīpikā contains the description of sex practices such as vajroli. What is the role of these practices in yoga? Are they useful?

Let us first look at the role of sex and non-attachment in the base text on yoga, the Yoga Sūtra. The Yoga Sūtra is not a text for celibates. While brahmacarya or control over all the senses, particularly the urge for sex, presented as one of the niyama-s, that does not mean celibacy. The definition depends on the situation in one's life. The requirement is not for celibacy *per se*, but ethical and balanced engagement in all activities, including sex, so that it fosters the state of sattva (calm, clear, pleasant).

The Yoga Sūtra presents the psychological facts. We all understand that sensory pleasures are not synonymous with contentment. Sensory pleasure is excitatory and temporary. Contentment is basal and lasting.

Hedonism, unrestrained sensory enjoyment, is an unreliable pathway to a state of calmness and stability because of the nature of the mind and the senses; the more we enjoy food and sex, the harder it is to let go of them. But we do need to learn to disengage with ease from these pleasures without pain and regret. After all, we cannot experience them always (because of energy, time, life situations, body constraints, age and more). If we do not learn how to engage in ethical and balanced sensory enjoyment, with limits, it will become an addiction, a pathology. This insight is also quite well enunciated in other ancient philosophies around the world such as stoicism.

Hence, to find a peaceful, sattva-dominant state of mind and body, we have to gradually moderate our attachment to the pleasures of the senses and cultivate a feeling of equanimity toward sensory experiences.

Note carefully here that there is no rejection of food or sex—only balance. In the case of sex, for a monk, this translates to celibacy. For a person in a relationship, this translates to being within the boundaries and expectations of that relationship. The keys are ethics and balance, without which ill-health in body and mind are likely.

Acknowledging these points, let us ask of the tantric sex practices, "How will these lead to a sattva-dominant state of mind and body?"

Finding long term contentment and steadiness of mind through unbridled hedonistic enjoyment, of sex, food or other sensory pleasures, is not rationally possible. Instead, the tantric sex practices seek to ritualize these sensory experiences. Ritualizing any strong sensory attachment in the form of worship is something that should be done with immense care. There is a great likelihood that such a practice will result in a rajas- or tamas-dominant state. In other words, it often results in addiction or agitation rather than calmness.

Why not, for instance, propose that we reduce sugar cravings by creating rituals and meditation around sweets as the principal practice? We understand that it is quite unlikely to work, just as ritualizing the practice of drinking alcohol is not a reliable way to control a drinking habit. To reduce sugar cravings, mindfulness and even simple rituals around the act of eating can be part of the approach. But these should be done in small steps, working with less addictive foods first, not with sweets.

Otherwise, the strength of habit and unconscious tendencies in the mind can easily carry one away into reliving the sensory experience and being increasingly addicted to it.

A more intelligent and effective pathway of dealing with craving for sweets would be through mindful movement, breathing, stress reduction, self-compassion etc. and gradual avoidance of the problematic stimulus (i.e. sweets)! Once the mind and senses are more stable, gradual exposure to sweets with mindfulness and perhaps in a structured or ritualized context can help the person deal with their craving.

The idea of using the five Ms (*panca ma-kāra sādhana*—five Sanskrit words starting with "M" including meat, alcohol, sex etc.) in some of the tantric texts is an offshoot of the psychology that these desires can be managed by making them ritual and symbolic. At least, it is symbolic in the clearer texts, but came to be treated literally in some others.

Rajas- and tamas-dominant states are easy to attain. Sattva-adominant states have to be earned. It is highly unlikely that an individual will experience increasing sattva through practices centered on a strong sensory stimulus with powerful natural attachments like food, sex, or alcohol.

Indulging in these is unlikely to remove the desire for them, even if done ritually. It is theoretically possible, but only in a very narrow set of circumstances for a practitioner who already has a strong will and steady mind. Without a strong will and steady mind, such practices are understandably problematic. And if one has a strong will and steady mind, why do these practices? You likely do not need them. This is the rational paradox.

That is why, on the surface, some of the esoteric practices look attractive. However, a simple reason why they have not been popular traditionally is not because they were "secret" and "powerful," but because they rarely work and are likely to deceive practitioners into restless and disturbed states of mind, rather than leaving them calm and clear. Mostly, the promise they make is of hedonism leading to calmness because it is ritualized. This is, for most people, a case of expecting to eat one's cake and have it too; very unlikely given how the body and mind function.

Neither a crash diet nor binge eating will lead to health and well-being in body or mind in the long run though they make us feel better for a while. Similarly, neither suppressing and rejecting sex nor worshipping it will leave us feeling better in body or mind in the long run. To find sattva or well-being, we have to find a nuanced path of balance.

There is another claim surrounding these tantric sex practices. Namely, that the energy of sex is powerful, and it can be "harnessed" to accelerate spiritual transformation. The problem with such descriptions in these texts is the usual lack of clarity on how that is supposed to be achieved, and the absence of any sound explanation of the body-mind pathways that are supposed to support such a process.

If one is looking for powerful forces in the body and mind, the greatest is already foundational to haṭha-yoga and is harnessed by the yogi: it is none other than breathing.

Not just sex, but breathing, movement, food, basic emotions (fear, anger, love) are all powerful foundations for the behavior of the body and mind. There is nothing particularly mystic about any of them more than the other, or about sex alone in particular, that will serve as a platform for self-transformation. They are all very important.

Krishnamacharya's perspective was that some of the yogis of the Nāth sects, such as Matsyendrānatha and Gorakshānatha, were not of the left-handed school, and the tantric sex practices we see in this text are later confusions. Krishnamacharya was not critical of the Nāth yogis, but of Svātmārāma.

Khecarī Mudrā

Khecarī mudrā is an interesting practice. There are two khecarī mudrā practices in this text, one each in Chapters III and IV respectively. The khecarī mudrā in Chapter III is not recommended—it involves cutting the frenulum of the tongue and folding it backward to press on the underside of the palate. The khecarī mudrā in Chapter IV is acceptable.

The concept of the practice of khecarī mudrā is to stimulate nerve centers in the posterior of the palate. This will create an altered body-mind connection and a reduction in body sensation, a sort of a shortcut to the same experience (reduction in body sensation and activity) that the yogi is aiming for through all the other practices as noted above.

By itself, this practice will not create the desired transformation in body-mind habits, but it is not unsound when done within the framework of the other preparations and practices of yoga.

Kriyā-s or Cleansing Techniques

The Haṭha Yoga Pradīpikā mentions six kriyā-s or cleansing techniques. The purpose of these practices is to make the body light and remove residual matter from the gastrointestinal tract, especially the colon, to the extent possible.

Ayurveda deals with similar techniques under the heading of *pañcakarma*. However, the techniques are nuanced in ayurveda, whereas, these kriyā-s are a blunt instrument.

Note that the text itself points out that these are not to be done unless one has excess fat or kapha. Those whose bodies are not afflicted with excess fat or kapha are not good candidates for these kriyā-s; they may result in ill-health.

Krishnamacharya was of the view that cleansing should largely be taken care of by light diet, and effective āsana and prāṇāyāma. It should not be necessary to do too much of the kriyā-s. If required, pañcakarma in accordance with the approach of ayurveda is the much better option.

Pathways in the Haṭha Yoga Pradīpikā and Gheraṇḍa Samhitā

The Gheraṇḍa Samhitā follows this structure in the haṭha-yoga practices:

- kriyā-s (ghata śodhana or cleansing the body)
- āsana-s: 32
- mudrā-s: 25
- pratyāhāra
- prāṇāyāma

The Haṭha Yoga Pradīpikā follows this order:

- āsana-s: 11 + 4
- prāṇāyāma: nāḍīśodhana + 8
- mudrā-s: 10
- nādānusandhāna

Studying the Haṭha Yoga Pradīpikā with Krishnamacharya

My studies with my teacher, the pioneering yogi, Sri Krishnamacharya, on the Haṭha Yoga Pradīpikā began on 17 July 1976. I recall this because I see the exact date in my notes from the first class. I have preserved all the notes I took down in my nearly two decades of studies with Krishnamacharya. Generally, all my studies with him used to take place in his room, perhaps 10x15 feet. He used to stay in the same room; his bed and a chair were part of the room's furniture, and a carpet for his āsana practice.

My studies on the Haṭha Yoga Pradīpikā took place in two phases. I studied the first two chapters starting in 1976, and Krishnamacharya stopped in the middle of the third chapter. He declined to teach further, opining that the latter portions were unnecessary.

In 1980, I began studying the Gheraṇḍa Samhitā and after some persuasion, Krishnamacharya agreed to take me through the rest of the Haṭha Yoga Pradīpikā as well.

Krishnamacharya was unique in his practice, knowledge, and experience in haṭha-yoga. I studied the Haṭha Yoga Pradīpikā and Gheraṇḍa Samhitā entirely privately with Krishnamacharya, one to one. I do not know if Krishnamacharya shared what he taught me on these topics with any of his other students. This is one more reason why I want to make his views and insights on this topic available to everyone.

Krishnamacharya's Writings and Haṭha-Yoga

In 1934, Krishnamacharya wrote a book titled the *Yoga Makaranda* ("Honey of Yoga"). The book was apparently authored in just a couple of nights (according to his wife), at the behest of the Maharaja of Mysore.

In that book, Krishnamacharya simply reproduces the description of the mudrā-s and their benefits from the Gheraṇḍa Samhitā. He leaves out five of the twenty-five, thus describing twenty mudrā-s. The five mudrā-s he leaves are out are meditation on the five elements (*pancabhūta-dhāraṇā*). These are strictly not mudrā-s but *siddhis* (special results) based on prāṇāyāma. They are described in the Yoga Yājñavalkya, VIII.15-25.

The Yoga Makaranda also contains:

- exaggerations similar to the older texts which he would dismiss in his classes;
- dṛṣṭi-s (focusing the gaze) he would not recommend (such as focusing the gaze between the eyebrows in mahāmudrā);
- breathing practices that he would not recommend (some practices based on holding the breath after inhalation);

- extreme āsana-s such as dvipāda-śīrṣāsana which he rarely taught later (relating them to kuṇḍalinī arousal, which he would present differently in his classes).

The explanation for this is probably that he simply put in whatever was in the older texts, getting the book out in a hurry, and the need to popularize yoga in those days. The Yoga Makaranda is not representative of Krishnamacharya's teachings in several respects as it glosses over the critical thinking and insight that usually characterized his classes on haṭha-yoga.

His slightly later book, *Yogāsanagalu,* is more balanced and somewhat more reflective of his teachings, but is still substantially incomplete.

In a video taken of Krishnamacharya in 1938, he demonstrates very slow movement, and mainly variations of inversion and prāṇāyāma with bandhas. This would characterize his presentation on these topics later, pointing out that this is enough, and the other mudrā-s and practices are not necessary.

Practice Pathway of Classical Haṭha-Yoga

Krishnamacharya's Guidelines

Here is a summary of Krishnamacharya's guidelines on the step-wise practice of classical haṭha-yoga.

1. Prepare the body and breathing with deep, long breathing and a well-rounded āsana practice according to fitness and capacity.
2. Cultivate inner or subtle body awareness gradually with the breathing.
3. Learn to increase the pause after exhalation.
4. Practice the three bandha-s (mūla, jalandhara, uḍḍīyāna) in simple āsana-s (taḍāga mudrā, bridge pose, chair pose).
5. Appreciate the feeling of the bandha-s/mudrā-s in the practice.
6. Practice the bandha-s in shoulderstand and headstand and deepen that awareness.
7. Practice nāḍīśodhana and basic prāṇāyāma-s.
8. Do mahāmudrā (with the three bandha-s).
9. Bring the bandha-s into prāṇāyāma and practice them for longer durations, deepening the subtle inner body experience from that practice.
10. Merge this with other meditations gradually as required.

Example Foundations for Bandha-s and Mudrā-s

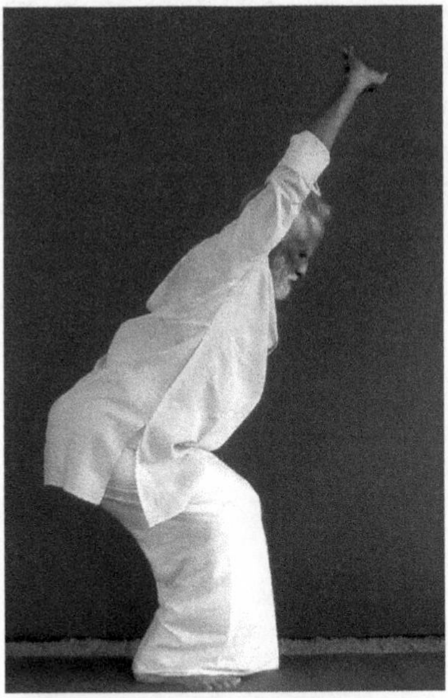

ardha utkaṭāsana

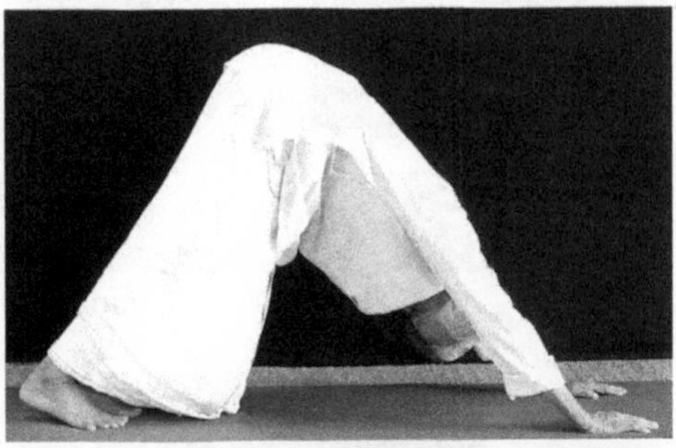

adhomukhaśvānāsana

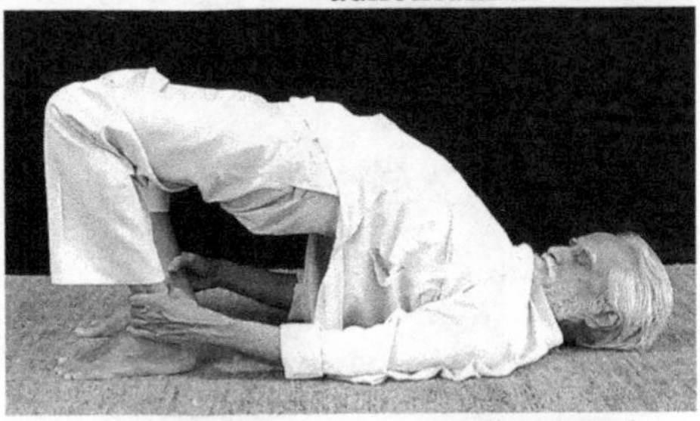

dvipādapīṭhaṁ

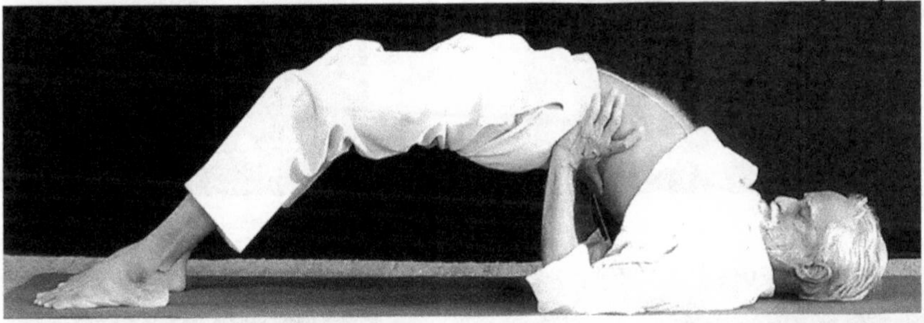

uttāna mayūrāsana

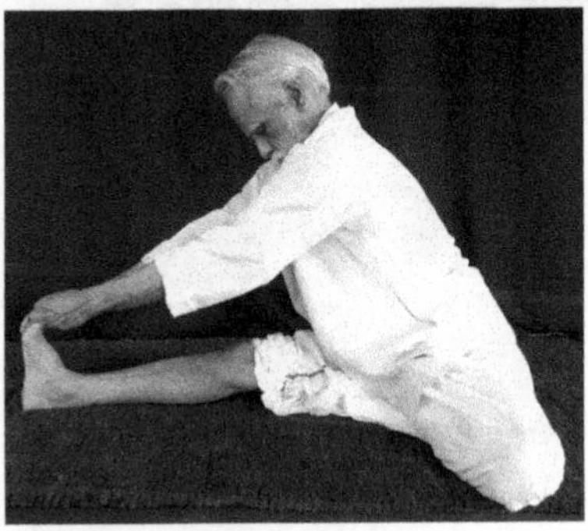

mahāmudrā

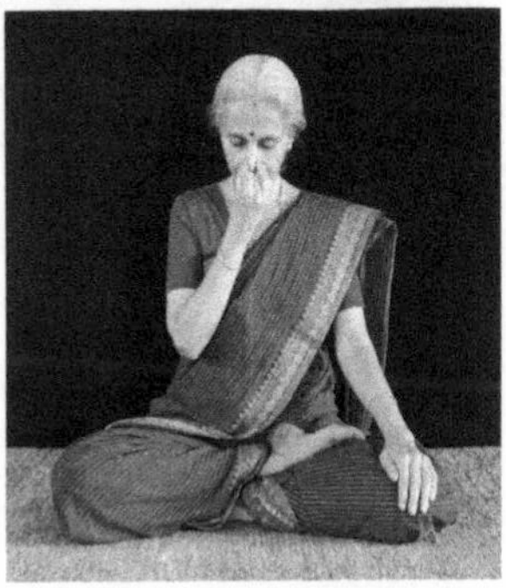

prāṇāyāma

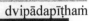

Example Practices with Bandha-s and Mudrā-s

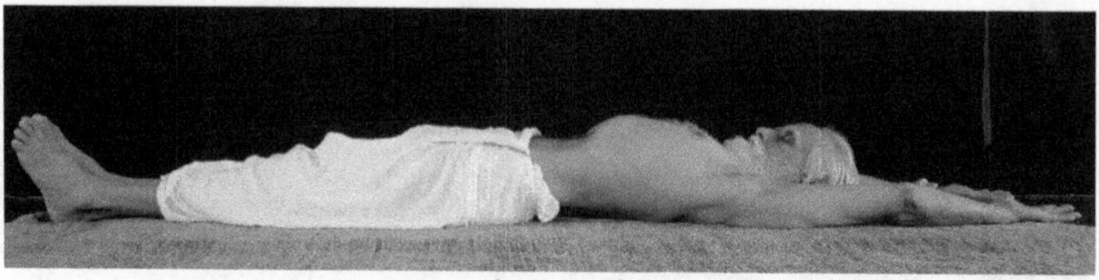

taḍāga mudrā

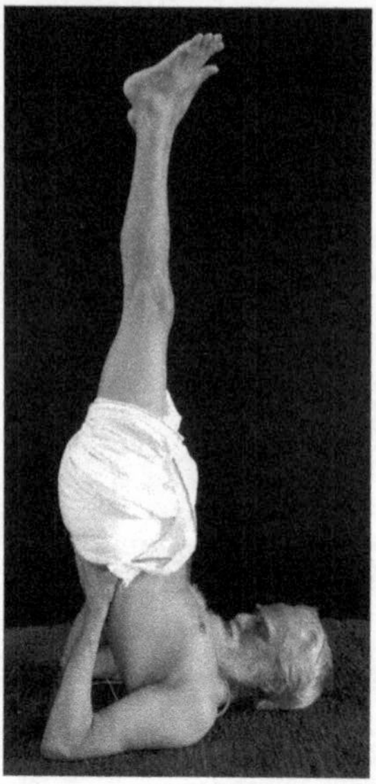

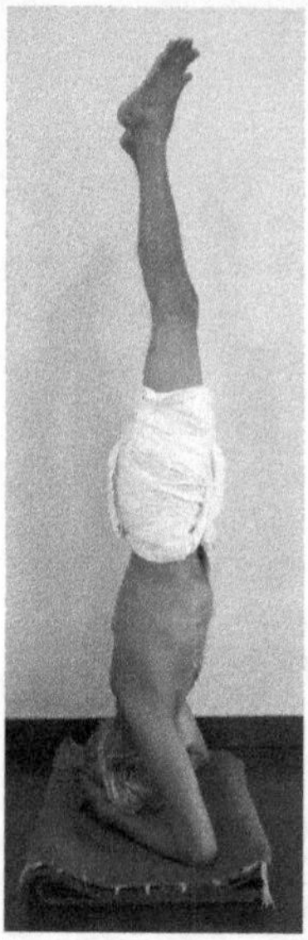

viparītakaraṇi mudrā

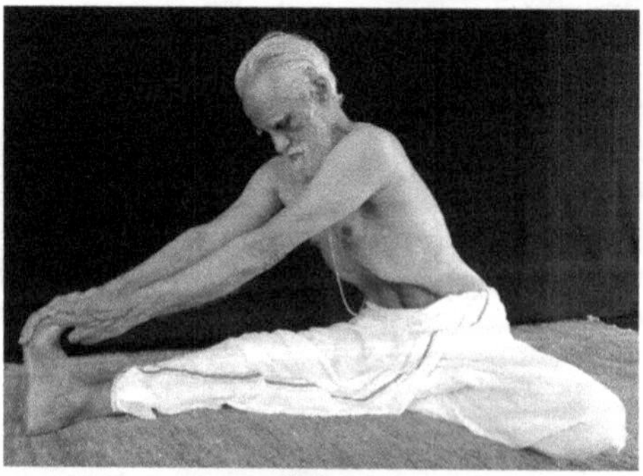

mahāmudrā

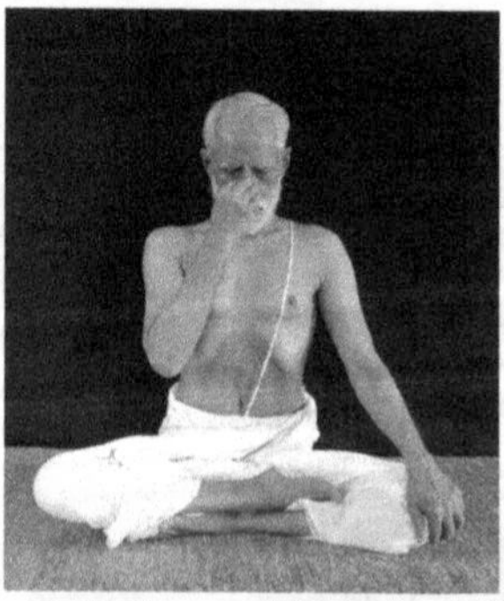

prāṇāyāma with the bandha-s

Concise Summary of the Text

Chapter I

1-16: Prayer. Prerequisites for haṭha-yoga and rāja-yoga. Haṭha-yoga teachers. Haṭha-yoga as the foundation for other yogas. Environment and place for practicing haṭha-yoga. Factors responsible for success and failure in haṭha-yoga.

17-32: Āsana-s approved by rāja-yogis and haṭha-yogis. List of eleven āsana-s and their benefits.

33-54: Four seated āsana-s for prāṇāyāma and meditation and their benefits.

55-67: The four steps of haṭha-yoga. Diet: what should be eaten, what should not be eaten. There are no age restrictions to practicing haṭha-yoga. Success is dependent on effort.

Chapter II

1-3: Why practice prāṇāyāma? Breath and mind connection.

4-6: The need to cleanse the nāḍī-s to attain samādhi.

7-10: The practice of nāḍīśodhana prāṇāyāma.

11-14: Repetitions of prāṇāyāma-s. Three stages of prāṇāyāma. Food guidelines.

15-20: Cautions about improper practice. How appropriate practice can lead to benefits.

21-37: Kriyā-s: list, methodology, benefits.

38-43: Importance of practicing prāṇāyāma with bandha-s and their benefits.

44-71: Eight types of prāṇāyāma and their benefits.

72-74: Kevala-kumbhaka.

75-78: Haṭha-yoga and rāja-yoga.

Chapter III

Chapter III contains a description of the ten mudrā-s and how to practice them. Several of these mudrā-s are found in other texts too. We have included below the list of these mudrā-s from the Gheraṇḍa Saṁhitā.

Number	Haṭha Yoga Pradīpikā	Mudrā	Gheraṇḍa Saṁhitā
	1-9	Introduction	1-5
1	10-18	Mahāmudrā	6-8
2	19-25	Mahāvedha	21-24
3	26-31	Mahābandha	18-20
4	32-54	Khecarī	25-32
5	55-60	Uḍḍīyāna-bandha	10-11
6	61-69	Mūla-bandha	14-17
7	70-76	Jālandhara-bandha	12-13
8	77-82	Viparītakaraṇī	33-36
9	83-91 92-95 96-103	Vajrolī Amarolī Sahajolī	-
10	104-130	Śakti-cālana	49-60

Chapter IV

1-14: Description and praise of samādhi (raja-yoga).

15-30: The relation between mind and prāṇa.

31-42: Description of laya and the means to it.

43-48: Khecarī mudrā—its practice and its result (yoga-nidrā).

54-64: Non-dualism.

65-81: Attainment of samādhi and nāda by piercing the cakras through prāṇāyāma (four stages).

82-103: Nādānusandhāna or feeling the inner sound or sensation, from gross to subtle.

104-115: Praise.

Chapter I

Chapter I: Detailed Summary

1-2: Salutation to guru and the Divine.

2-3: The purpose of haṭha-yoga is to lead to rāja-yoga. Everyone needs haṭha-yoga.

4: The guru pathway of Svātmārāma (Matsyendranātha and Gorakṣanātha).

5-9: List of haṭha-yogis.

10: Haṭha-yoga is the foundation of removing all suffering.

11: Need to maintain secrecy in the practice.

12-13: Ideal surroundings for the practice.

14: Qualities of the aspirant for a successful outcome.

15: Reasons why the practices of haṭha-yoga will fail.

16: Reasons why the practices of haṭha-yoga will succeed.

17: Āsana is the first limb of haṭha-yoga. Benefit or expected result of āsana.

18: Introduction to āsana-s to be described.

19: Svastikāsana

20: Gomukhāsana

21: Vīrāsana

22: Kūrmāsana

23: Kukkuṭāsana

24: Uttāna-kūrmāsana

25: Dhanurāsana

26: Matsyendrāsana

27: Benefits of matsyendrāsana.

28: Paścimatānāsana

29: Benefits of paścimatānāsana.

30: Mayūrāsana

31: Benefits of mayūrāsana.

32: Śavāsana

33-34: Four particularly important āsana-s will now be described.

35-37: Siddhāsana

38-43: Benefits and praise of siddhāsana.

44-49: Benefits and praise of padmāsana.

50-52: Benefits and praise of simhāsana.

53-54: Benefits and praise of bhadrāsana.

55: Prāṇāyāma follows effortless āsana.

56: Pathway (krama) of haṭha-yoga.

57: How long will it take?

58: Moderation in diet.

59-60: Foods to avoid.

61: Activities to avoid.

62-63: Foods to be consumed.

64: Everyone can practice yoga.

65-66: Importance of practice for success in yoga.

67: Haṭha-yoga should be practiced until rāja-yoga is established.

Chapter I: Translation

अथ हठयोगप्रदीपिका।
श्रीआदिनाथाय नमोऽस्तु तस्मै येनोपदिष्टा हठयोगविद्या ।
विभ्राजते प्रोन्नतराजयोगमारोढुमिच्छोरधिरोहिणीव ॥ १ ॥

atha haṭhayogapradīpikā |
śrīādināthāya namo'stu tasmai yenopadiṣṭā haṭhayogavidyā |
vibhrājate pronnatarājayogamāroḍhumicchoradhirohiṇīva ||1||

I.1: Salutations to Śrī Ādinātha who taught the knowledge (vidyā) of haṭha-yoga which is like a ladder to those who wish to attain the lofty rāja-yoga.

[Krishnamacharya] "Ādinātha" could refer to Śiva or to Viṣṇu according to the commentary of Brahmānanda. The word "haṭha" consists of two parts, *ha* and *ṭha*. The two parts are traditionally connected with the meaning or symbology like this:

ha: piṅgalā, sun, prāṇa, inhale.

ṭha: iḍā, moon, apāna, exhale.

The traditional concept is to unite or balance these two.

This is where we find the statement, in the commentary, that haṭha-yoga is prāṇāyāma. The particular prāṇāyāma referred to here is the kevala-kumbhaka or fourth (caturtha) prāṇāyāma of the Yoga Sūtra (II.51: bāhya-ābhyantara-viṣaya-ākṣepī caturthaḥ)

The Bhagavad Gitā (IV.29) refers to this prāṇāyāma as well, and all the major commentators (ācārya-s) agree on this.

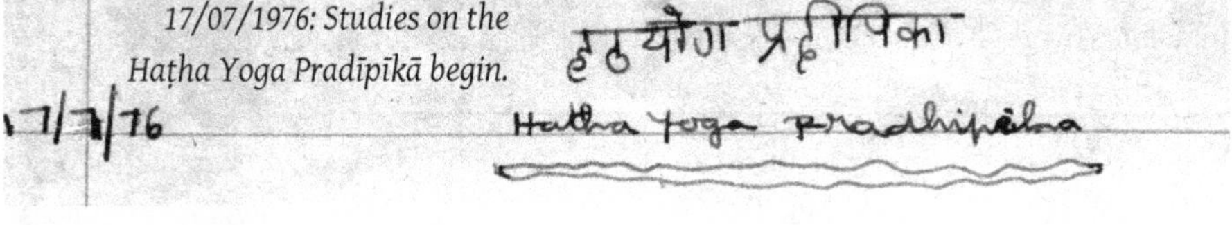

17/07/1976: Studies on the Haṭha Yoga Pradīpikā begin.

प्रणम्य श्रीगुरुं नाथं स्वात्मारामेण योगिना ।
केवलं राजयोगाय हठविद्योपदिश्यते ॥ २ ॥

praṇamya śrīguruṁ nāthaṁ svātmārāmeṇa yoginā |
kevalaṁ rājayogāya haṭhavidyopadiśyate ||2||

I.2: Svātmārāma yogi after saluting his lord and guru, presents the knowledge (vidyā) of haṭha-yoga only for the sake of [attaining] rāja-yoga.

भ्रान्त्या बहुमतध्वान्ते राजयोगमजानताम् ।
हठप्रदीपिकां धत्ते स्वात्मारामः कृपाकरः ॥ ३ ॥

bhrāntyā bahumatadhvānte rājayogamajānatām |
haṭhapradīpikāṁ dhatte svātmārāmaḥ kṛpākaraḥ ||3||

I.3: For those who are ignorant of rāja-yoga and are confused in the darkness of conflicting doctrines, the compassionate Svātmārāma offers the light of the knowledge of haṭha-yoga.

[Krishnamacharya] used to mention this quotation: "śarīram ādyaṁ khalu dharma-sādhanam." "The body is the path to dharma (useful or ethical action)."

Physical health is required for achieving any goals, spiritual or material, and haṭha-yoga is the pathway that can give that. This text talks about haṭha-yoga and laya-yoga, which leads to rāja-yoga. Mantra-yoga is not explained in this text, and that is the doctrine referred to here which may lead to confusion.

हठविद्यां हि मत्स्येन्द्रगोरक्षाद्या विजानते ।
स्वात्मारामोऽथवा योगी जानीते तत्प्रसादतः ॥ ४ ॥

haṭhavidyāṁ hi matsyendragorakṣādyā vijānate |
svātmārāmo'thavā yogī jānīte tatprasādataḥ ||4||

I.4: Matsyendra, Gorakṣa, and others are well versed in the knowledge of haṭha-yoga. By their grace, yogi Svātmārāma also learned it.

[Krishnamacharya] The Nātha yogis (Matsyendranātha, Gorakṣanātha etc.) are śaivite by tradition (practicing devotion to the deity Śiva).

The word "grace" here can be misleading. The Sanskrit word *prasāda* actually means calm clarity of the mind. This appears in the Yoga Sūtra in several key places too. One attains success not merely by being in the tradition of a teacher, but by understanding and practicing the teachings until the mind is clear and steady.

श्रीआदिनाथमत्स्येन्द्रशाबरानन्दभैरवाः ।
चौरङ्गीमीनगोरक्षविरूपाक्षबिलेशयाः ॥५॥
मन्थानो भैरवो योगी सिद्धिर्बुद्धश्च कन्थडिः ।
कोरण्टकः सुरानन्दः सिद्धपादश्च चर्पटिः ॥६॥
कानेरी पूज्यपादश्च नित्यनाथो निरञ्जनः ।
कपाली बिन्दुनाथश्च काकचण्डीश्वराह्वयः ॥७॥
अल्लामः प्रभुदेवश्च घोडाचोली च टिण्टिणिः ।
भानुकी नारदेवश्च खण्डः कापालिकस्तथा ॥८॥
इत्यादयो महासिद्धा हठयोगप्रभावतः ।
खण्डयित्वा कालदण्डं ब्रह्माण्डे विचरन्ति ते ॥९॥

śrīādināthamatsyendraśābarānandabhairavāḥ |
cauraṅgīmīnagorakṣavirūpākṣabileśayāḥ ||5||

manthāno bhairavo yogī siddhirbuddhaśca kanthaḍiḥ |
koraṇṭakaḥ surānandaḥ siddhapādaśca carpaṭiḥ ||6||

kānerī pūjyapādaśca nityanātho nirañjanaḥ |
kapālī bindunāthaśca kākacaṇḍīśvarāhvayaḥ ||7||

allāmaḥ prabhudevaśca ghoḍācolī ca ṭiṇṭiṇiḥ |
bhānukī nāradevaśca khaṇḍaḥ kāpālikastathā ||8||

ityādayo mahāsiddhā haṭhayogaprabhāvataḥ |
khaṇḍayitvā kāladaṇḍaṁ brahmāṇḍe vicaranti te ||9||

I.5-9: Śrīādinātha, Matsyendra, Śābara, Ānandabhairava, Cauraṅgī, Mīna, Gorakṣa, Virūpākṣa, Bileśaya, Manthāna, Bhairava, Siddhi, Buddha, Kanthaḍi, Koraṇṭaka, Surānanda, Siddhapāda, Carpaṭi, Kānerī, Pūjyapāda, Nityanātha, Nirañjana, Kapālī, Bindunātha, Kākacaṇḍīśvara, Allāma, Prabhudeva, Ghoḍācolī, Ṭiṇṭiṇi, Bhānukī, Nāradeva, Khaṇḍaḥ, Kāpālika and many other great adepts (siddha-s), having conquered time through the power of haṭha-yoga, move about this universe.

[Krishnamacharya] Krishnamacharya used to acknowledge and praise Matsyendranātha and Gorakṣanātha. He did not, however, approve of the Kāpalika-s.

While the tāntrics are also approved of in the Yoga Yājñavalkya, not all tāntrics mentioned in that text are Kāpalika-s or associated with left-handed tāntric practices. The latter is what Krishnamacharya used to take exception to.

अशेषतापतप्तानां समाश्रयमठो हठः ।
अशेषयोगयुक्तानामाधारकमठो हठः ॥१०॥

aśeṣatāpataptānāṁ samāśrayamaṭho haṭhaḥ |
aśeṣayogayuktānāmādhārakamaṭho haṭhaḥ ||10||

I.10: Haṭha-yoga is a sheltering monastery for those scorched by all the [three] kinds of suffering. Haṭha-yoga is a foundational support for those who are engaged in the practice of different kinds of yoga.

[Krishnamacharya] The three kinds of suffering are those arising from natural causes, from other living beings, and from oneself. Another way of classifying suffering is that arising from the body, and from the mind. Since haṭha-yoga is crucial for physical well-being, it is essential for removing bodily suffering. Bodily suffering is in turn a foundation for psychological suffering, hence haṭha-yoga is a support for removing all suffering.

हठविद्या परं गोप्या योगिना सिद्धिमिच्छता ।
भवेद् वीर्यवती गुप्ता निर्वीर्या तु प्रकाशिता ॥११॥

haṭhavidyā paraṁ gopyā yoginā siddhimicchatā |
bhaved vīryavatī guptā nirvīryā tu prakāśitā ||11||

I.11: The yogi who is desirous of attaining success (siddhi), should keep the knowledge of haṭha-yoga very secret. It will be potent when it is kept secret and ineffective when publicly revealed.

सुराज्ये धार्मिके देशे सुभिक्षे निरूपद्रवे ।
धनुःप्रमाणपर्यन्तं शिलाग्निजलवर्जिते ।
एकान्ते मठिकामध्ये स्थातव्यं हठयोगिना ॥१२॥

surājye dhārmike deśe subhikṣe nirūpadrave |
dhanuḥ pramāṇaparyantaṁ śilāgnijalavarjite |
ekānte maṭhikāmadhye sthātavyaṁ haṭhayoginā ||12||

I.12: One who practices haṭha-yoga should live alone in a small monastery (maṭha), situated a bow's length away from rocks, water, and fire, in a virtuous, well-ruled kingdom which is prosperous and free of disturbances.

अल्पद्वारमरन्ध्रगर्तविवरं नात्युच्चनीचायतं
सम्यग्गोमयसान्द्रलिप्तममलं निःशेषजन्तूज्झितम्।
बाह्ये मण्डपवेदिकूपरुचिरं प्राकारसंवेष्टितं
प्रोक्तं योगमठस्य लक्षणमिदं सिद्धैर्हठाभ्यासिभिः ॥ १३ ॥

alpadvāramarandhragartavivaraṁ nātyuccanīcāyataṁ
samyaggomayasāndraliptamamalaṁ niḥśeṣajantūjjhitam|
bāhye maṇḍapavedikūparuciraṁ prākārasaṁveṣṭitaṁ
proktaṁ yogamaṭhasya lakṣaṇamidaṁ siddhairhaṭhābhyāsibhiḥ||13||

I.13: The monastery (maṭha) should have a small door, without any windows. It should be level, without any holes in the floor. It should not be too high, too low, or too long. It should be well smeared with cow dung and kept clean, free from all insects. Outside it should be beautiful with a small hall (maṇḍapa), a raised seat and a well, and surrounded by a wall. These are the characteristics of a yoga maṭha as laid down by the adepts (siddha-s) who have practiced haṭha-yoga.

[Krishnamacharya] Chapter 5 of the Yoga Yājñavalkya (22 verses) describes in detail the surroundings conducive to the practice of yoga.

एवंविधे मठे स्थित्वा सर्वचिन्ताविवर्जितः ।
गुरूपदिष्टमार्गेण योगमेव सदाभ्यसेत् ॥ १४ ॥

evaṁvidhe maṭhe sthitvā sarvacintāvivarjitaḥ |
gurūpadiṣṭamārgeṇa yogameva sadābhyaset ||14||

I.14: Living in such a monastery, with a mind free of all worries, the yogi should practice yoga all the time as taught by his guru.

[Krishnamacharya] There is no description here for inducing particular discomfort to the body or being in surroundings that create physical strain like excessive heat or cold.

अत्याहारः प्रयासश्च प्रजल्पो नियमग्रहः ।
जनसङ्गश्च लौल्यं च षड्भिर्योगो विनश्यति ॥ १५ ॥

atyāhāraḥ prayāsaśca prajalpo niyamagrahaḥ |
janasaṅgaśca laulyaṁ ca ṣaḍbhiryogo vinaśyati ||15||

I.15: Yoga fails due to six causes: over-eating, over-exertion, excessive talk, observance of inappropriate disciplines, promiscuous company, and unsteadiness.

[Krishnamacharya] used to emphasize the importance of eating in moderation, for the successful practice of haṭha-yoga. Regarding over-exertion, as an example, in I.61 excessive sun salutation (sūryanamaskāra) is considered to induce needless physical discomfort.

उत्साहात् साहसात् धैर्यात् तत्त्वज्ञानाच्च निश्चयात् ।
जनसङ्गपरित्यागात् षड्भिर्योगः प्रसिध्यति ॥ १६ ॥

utsāhāt sāhasāt dhairyāt tattvajñānācca niścayāt |
janasaṅgaparityāgāt ṣaḍbhiryogaḥ prasiddhyati ||16||

I.16: Yoga succeeds through the following six factors: zeal, discriminative determination, courage, true knowledge, conviction, and renunciation of the company of (inappropriate) people.

[Krishnamacharya] The word "sāhasa" means to put in effort knowing one's capacity. "True knowledge" is to understand the elements of yoga accurately.

अथ आसनम् ।
हठस्य प्रथमाङ्गत्वादासनं पूर्वमुच्यते ।
कुर्यात्तदासनं स्थैर्यमारोग्यं चाङ्गलाघवम् ॥ १७ ॥

haṭhasya prathamāṅgatvādāsanaṁ pūrvamucyate |
kuryāttadāsanaṁ sthairyamārogyaṁ cāṅgalāghavam ||17||

Now āsana [is described].

I.17: Āsana-s are spoken of in the first place, as they are the first component of haṭha-yoga. Āsana-s bring about steadiness, lightness of limbs, and freedom from illness.

[Krishnamacharya] This text begins haṭha-yoga with the practice of āsana-s. There are versions of this text with yama-s and niyama-s listed before this verse. The yama-s and niyama-s appear to be borrowed from the Yoga Yājñavalkya (they are practically identical). The commentary of Brahmānanda does not mention the verses on the yama-s and niyama-s.

Krishnamacharya was critical of the text at this point as it does not explicitly start with the yama-s and niyama-s. Āsana-s do not become yoga unless when done with the yama-s and niyama-s.

The last four limbs of Patañjali's yoga (pratyāhāra, dhāraṇā, dhyāna, samādhi), the commentator holds, arise through the practice of nādānusandhāna itself.

Steadiness here is the reduction of restlessness or rajas in both body and mind. Lightness of the body is reduction of the heaviness in the body, or the quality of tamas. When both are achieved, the quality of balance or sattva arises, and there is good health in body and greater mental clarity.

This section lists eleven āsana-s, and the next section lists four āsana-s. The description, like in other traditional texts, is terse and incomplete. Also, the names of āsana-s are not always consistent across texts. The expectation is that these are to be learned practically from a teacher, of course.

Other texts including the Gheraṇḍa Saṁhitā present more āsana-s.

वसिष्ठाद्यैश्च मुनिभिर्मत्स्येन्द्राद्यैश्च योगिभिः ।
अङ्गीकृतान्यासनानि कथ्यन्ते कानिचिन्मया ॥१८॥

vasiṣṭhādyaiśca munibhirmatsyendrādyaiśca yogibhiḥ |
aṅgīkṛtānyāsanāni kathyante kānicinmayā ||18||

I.18: I shall proceed to describe some of the āsana-s considered appropriate by such sages as Vasiṣṭha and yogis such as Matsyendra.

[Krishnamacharya] Brahmānanda's commentary adds Yājñavalkya to the list of such sages.

जानूर्वोरन्तरे सम्यक्कृत्वा पादतले उभे ।
ऋजुकायः समासीनः स्वस्तिकं तत् प्रचक्षते ॥१९॥

jānūrvorantare samyakkṛtvā pādatale ubhe |
ṛjukāyaḥ samāsīnaḥ svastikaṁ tat pracakṣate ||19||

I.19: Having placed correctly, the soles of the feet between the thighs and the knees, one should sit balanced and straight. This is called svastikāsana.

सव्ये दक्षिणगुल्फं तु पृष्ठपार्श्वे नियोजयेत् ।
दक्षिणेऽपि तथा सव्यं गोमुखं गोमुखाकृति ॥२०॥

savye dakṣiṇagulphaṁ tu pṛṣṭhapārśve niyojayet |
dakṣiṇe'pi tathā savyaṁ gomukhaṁ gomukhākṛti ||20||

I.20: Place the right ankle next to the left buttock and the left ankle next to the right buttock. This is called gomukhāsana and it resembles the face of a cow.

[Krishnamacharya] was fond of the back salute in gomukhāsana.

एकं पादं तथैकस्मिन्वन्यसेदूरुणि स्थिरम्।
इतरस्मिन्स्तथा चोरुं वीरासनमितीरितम्॥२१॥

ekaṁ pādaṁ tathaikasminvanyasedūruṇi sthiram|
itarasminstathā coruṁ vīrāsanamitīritam||21||

1.21: Place one (the right) foot firmly on the other (left) thigh and the (right) thigh on the other (left) foot. This is called vīrāsana.

गुदं निरुध्य गुल्फाभ्यां व्युत्क्रमेण समाहितः ।
कूर्मासनं भवेदेतदिति योगविदो विदुः ॥२२॥

gudaṁ nirudhya gulphābhyāṁ vyutkrameṇa samāhitaḥ |
kūrmāsanaṁ bhavedetaditi yogavido viduḥ ||22||

1.22: Pressing the perineum with the ankles in the opposite direction, remain well poised. This is kūrmāsana, according to the yogis.

पद्मासनं तु संस्थाप्य जानूर्वोरन्तरे करौ ।
निवेश्य भूमौ संस्थाप्य व्योमस्थं कुक्कुटासनं ॥२३॥

padmāsanaṁ tu saṁsthāpya jānūrvorantare karau |
niveśya bhūmau saṁsthāpya vyomasthaṁ kukkuṭāsanam ||23||

1.23: Assuming padmāsana, insert the hands between the thighs and the knees. Placing them firmly on the ground, rise in the air (supported by the hands). This is kukkuṭāsana.

[Krishnamacharya] One should train further by walking on the hands in this āsana.

कुक्कुटासनबन्धस्थो दोर्भ्यां सम्बध्य कन्धराम् ।
भवेत्कूर्मवदुत्तान एतदुत्तान कूर्मकम् ॥ २४॥

kukkuṭāsanabandhastho dorbhyāṁ sambadhya kandharām |
bhavetkūrmavaduttāna etaduttānakūrmakam ||24||

1.24: Assuming kukkuṭāsana, wind the arms around the neck and lie on the back like a tortoise. This is called uttāna-kūrmāsana.

[Krishnamacharya] This is also called garbha-piṇḍāsana.

पादाङ्गुष्ठौ तु पाणिभ्यां गृहीत्वा श्रवणावधि ।
धनुराकर्षणं कुर्याद्धनुरासनमुच्यते ॥२५॥

pādāṅguṣṭhau tu pāṇibhyāṁ gṛhītvā śravaṇāvadhi |
dhanurākarṣaṇaṁ kuryāddhanurāsanamucyate ||25||

1.25: Taking hold of the big toes with the hands (keep one arm stretched in front and) draw (the other) up to the ear as if drawing a bow. This is called dhanurāsana.

[Krishnamacharya] This description is of the āsana that he used to call ākarṇa-dhanurāsana (to-the-ear bow pose).

वामोरुमूलार्पितदक्षपादं जानोर्बहिर्वेष्टितवामपादम् ।
प्रगृह्य तिष्ठेत् परिवर्तिताङ्गः श्रीमत्स्यनाथोदितमासनं स्यात् ॥२६॥

vāmorumūlārpitadakṣapādaṁ jānorbahirveṣṭitavāmapādam |
pragṛhya tiṣṭhet parivartitāṅgaḥ śrīmatsyanāthoditamāsanaṁ syāt ||26||

1.26: Placing the right foot at the base of the left thigh and left foot outside the right knee, take hold (of the right foot by the left hand and the left foot by the right hand) and remain with the body twisted (to the left). This is the āsana described as matsyendrāsana.

मत्स्येन्द्रपीठं जठरप्रदीप्तिं प्रचण्डरुग्मण्डलखण्डनास्त्रम् ।
अभ्यासतः कुण्डलिनीप्रबोधं चन्द्रस्थिरत्वं च ददाति पुंसाम् ॥२७॥

matsyendrapīṭhaṁ jaṭharapradīptiṁ pracaṇḍarugmaṇḍalakhaṇḍanāstram |
abhyāsataḥ kuṇḍalinīprabodhaṁ candrasthiratvaṁ ca dadāti puṁsām ||27||

1.27: This matsyendrāsana, which stimulates the gastric fire, is a weapon which destroys all the severe diseases of the body. With regular practice, it arouses the kuṇḍalinī and brings steadiness to the cooling nectar (candra) [flowing from above the palate] in men.

प्रसार्य पादौ भुवि दण्डरूपौ दोर्भ्यां पदाग्रद्वितयं गृहीत्वा ।
जानूपरि न्यस्तललाटदेशो वसेदिदं पश्चिमतानमाहुः ॥२८॥

prasārya pādau bhuvi daṇḍarūpau dorbhyāṁ padāgradvitayaṁ gṛhītvā |
jānūpari nyastalalāṭadeśo vasedidaṁ paścimatānamāhuḥ ||28||

1.28: Stretching out both the legs on the ground without bending them, hold the toes (soles) of the feet with the hands, place the forehead on the knees and stay there. This is called paścimatānāsana.

इति पश्चिमतानमासनाग्र्यं पवनं पश्चिमवाहिनं करोति ।
उदयं जठरानलस्य कुर्यादुदरे कार्श्यमरोगतां च पुंसाम् ॥२९॥

iti paścimatānamāsanāgryaṁ pavanaṁ paścimavāhinaṁ karoti |
udayaṁ jaṭharānalasya kuryādudare kārśyamarogatāṁ ca puṁsām ||29||

1.29: This paścimatānāsana, the most excellent among the āsana-s, makes the breath flow through the suṣumnā, stimulates the gastric fire, makes the abdomen slim, and removes all diseases.

[Krishnamacharya] Staying in paścimatānāsana, suspending the breath after exhalation, feeling the lower belly and pelvic floor (mūla) drawn in, is an important preparation for mahāmudrā.

धरामवष्टभ्य करद्वयेन तत्कूर्परस्थापितनाभिपार्श्वः ।
उच्चासनो दण्डवदुत्थितः खे मायूरमेतत्प्रवदन्ति पीठम् ॥३०॥

dharāmavaṣṭabhya karadvayena tatkūrparasthāpitanābhipārśvaḥ |
uccāsano daṇḍavadutthitaḥ khe māyūrametatpravadanti pīṭham ||30||

1.30: Place the hands firmly on the ground, place the elbows as a support on either side of the navel and raise the body like a straight rod, the feet above the ground in level with the head. This āsana is called mayūrāsana.

हरति सकलरोगानाशु गुल्मोदरादीनभिभवति च दोषानासनं श्रीमयूरम् ।
बहु कदशनभुक्तं भस्म कुर्यादशेषं जनयति जठराग्निं जारयेत् कालकूटम् ॥ ३१ ॥

harati sakalarogānāśu gulmodarādīnabhibhavati ca doṣānāsanaṁ śrīmayūram |
bahu kadaśanabhuktaṁ bhasma kuryādaśeṣaṁ janayati jaṭharāgniṁ jārayet kālakūṭam ||31||

1.31: Mayūrāsanā cures all diseases like enlargement of the glands, dropsy, and other stomach diseases, and overcomes the imbalance of the doṣas (vāta, pitta, and kapha). It reduces to ashes (i.e. enables digestion of) food eaten indiscriminately. It kindles the gastric fire and digests even the strongest of all poisons (kālakūṭa).

उत्तानं शववद्भूमौ शयनं तच्छवासनम् ।
शवासनं श्रान्तिहरं चित्तविश्रान्तिकारकम् ॥ ३२ ॥

uttānaṁ śavavadbhūmau śayanaṁ tacchavāsanaṁ |
śavāsanaṁ śrāntiharaṁ cittaviśrāntikārakam ||32||

1.32: Lying on the back on the ground like a corpse is śavāsana. Śavāsana removes fatigue and provides rest and peace to the mind.

चतुरशीत्यासनानि शिवेन कथितानि च ।
तेभ्यश्चतुष्कमादाय सारभूतं ब्रवीम्यहम् ॥ ३३ ॥

caturaśītyāsanāni śivena kathitāni ca |
tebhyaścatuṣkamādāya sārabhūtaṁ bravīmyaham ||33||

1.33: The āsana-s propounded by Śivā are eighty-four in number. I will describe four from them which are the quintessence.

सिद्धं पद्मं तथा सिंहं भद्रं वेति चतुष्टयम् ।
श्रेष्ठम् तत्रापि च सुखे तिष्ठेत् सिद्धासने सदा ॥३४॥

siddhaṁ padmaṁ tathā siṁhaṁ bhadraṁ veti catuṣṭayam |
śreṣṭhaṁ tatrāpi ca sukhe tiṣṭhet siddhāsane sadā ||34||

1.34: These four, siddhāsana, padmāsana, simhāsana, and bhadrāsana are the best. Of these, siddhāsana which is most comfortable must be practiced always.

[Krishnamacharya] These four āsana-s will be used for prāṇāyāma and the bandha-s. The principal focus is on reducing the drive for food and sex. The seated āsana-s are a pathway to that. The extensive praise of siddhāsana is because it helps control the sex urge physically.

तत्र सिद्धासनम् ।
योनिस्थानकमङ्घ्रिमूलघटितं कृत्वा दृढं विन्यसेन्मेण्ढ्रे पादमथैकमेव हृदये कृत्वा हनुं सुस्थिरम् ।
स्थाणुः संयमितेन्द्रियोऽचलदृशा पश्येद्भ्रुवोरन्तरं ह्येतन्मोक्षकपाटभेदजनकं सिद्धासनं प्रोच्यते ॥३५॥

tatra siddhāsanam |
yonisthānakamaṅghrimūlaghaṭitaṁ kṛtvā dṛḍhaṁ vinyasenmeṇḍhre
pādamathaikameva hṛdaye kṛtvā hanuṁ susthiram |
sthāṇuḥ saṁyamitendriyo'caladṛśā paśyedbhruvorantaraṁ
hyetanmokṣakapāṭabhedajanakaṁ siddhāsanaṁ procyate ||35||

Now siddhāsana [is described].

1.35: Press the perineum with the base of the heel and place the other heel firmly above the generative organ. Keep the chin firmly on the chest. Remain motionless with the senses under control and gaze at the spot between the eyebrows. This is called siddhāsana, which throws open the door to freedom.

[Krishnamacharya] This should be done with jālandhara-bandha, control of the senses, and with non-attachment. Being motionless should come from a feeling of being rooted to the earth.

मेण्ढ्रादुपरि विन्यस्य सव्यं गुल्फं तथोपरि ।
गुल्फान्तरं च निक्षिप्य सिद्धासनमिदं भवेत् ॥ ३६ ॥

meṇḍhrādupari vinyasya savyaṁ gulphaṁ tathopari |
gulphāntaraṁ ca nikṣipya siddhāsanamidaṁ bhavet ||36||

1.36: According to another view, placing the left ankle above the generative organ and placing the other ankle above it is called siddhāsana.

[Krishnamacharya] This involves pressing the genitals completely with both feet in a comfortable position. It can result in related triggers such as the urge to urinate and will not work unless the urge of sex is well controlled.

एतत्सिद्धासनं प्राहुरन्ये वज्रासनं विदुः ।
मुक्तासनं वदन्त्येके प्राहुर्गुप्तासनं परे ॥ ३७ ॥

etatsiddhāsanaṁ prāhuranye vajrāsanaṁ viduḥ |
muktāsanaṁ vadantyeke prāhurguptāsanaṁ pare ||37||

1.37: Some say this is siddhāsana, others know it as vajrāsana. Some call it as muktāsana and some others as guptāsana.

[Krishnamacharya] This is sometimes called vajrāsana because it makes the spine tall and strong (like a diamond); muktāsana because it leads to mokṣa or freedom; guptāsana because it protects or subdues the secret organs or the genitals.

यमेष्विव मिताहारमहिंसां नियमेष्विव ।
मुख्यं सर्वासनेष्वेकं सिद्धाः सिद्धासनं विदुः ॥ ३८ ॥

yameṣviva mitāhāramahiṁsāṁ niyameṣviva |
mukhyaṁ sarvāsaneṣvekaṁ siddhāḥ siddhāsanaṁ viduḥ ||38||

1.38: Just as a moderate diet is most important among the yama-s and non-harmfulness is most important among the niyama-s, the adepts (siddha-s) know that among the āsana-s it is guptāsana that is most important.

[Krishnamacharya] Note how moderation in diet is emphasized here. Because the practices of haṭha-yoga are principally physical, they are dependent on control over food intake.

चतुरशीतिपीठेषु सिद्धमेव सदाभ्यसेत् ।
द्वासप्ततिसहस्राणां नाडीनां मलशोधनम् ॥३९॥

caturaśītipīṭheṣu siddhameva sadābhyaset |
dvāsaptatisahasrāṇāṁ nāḍīnāṁ malaśodhanam ||39||

1.39: Of all the eighty-four asanas, one should always practice siddhāsana. It cleanses the 72,000 nāḍī-s.

आत्मध्यायी मिताहारी यावद्द्वादशवत्सरम् ।
सदा सिद्धासनाभ्यासात् योगी निष्पत्तिमाप्नुयात् ॥४०॥

ātmadhyāyī mitāhārī yāvaddvādaśavatsaram |
sadā siddhāsanābhyāsāt yogī niṣpattimāpnuyāt ||40||

1.40: The yogi who, meditating on the self and following a moderate diet, continually practices siddhāsana for twelve years attains samādhi.

[Krishnamacharya] Continually practicing siddhāsana means using it in prāṇāyāma, pūjā, and meditation. Siddhāsana is more for monks and those working toward celibacy because of the effect it has on sexual and reproductive function.

किमन्यैर्बहुभिः पीठैः सिद्धे सिद्धासने सति ।
प्राणानिले सावधाने बद्धे केवलकुम्भके ।
उत्पद्यते निरायासात् स्वयमेवोन्मनी कला ॥४१॥

kimanyairbahubhiḥ pīṭhaiḥ siddhe siddhāsane sati |
prāṇānile sāvadhāne baddhe kevalakumbhake |
utpadyate nirāyāsāt svayamevonmanī kalā ||41||

1.41: When one masters siddhāsana, of what use are the various other āsana-s? When prāṇa is restrained by the practice of spontaneous stillness of the breath (kevala-kumbhaka), absorption (unmanī-avasthā or samādhi) arises without any effort.

तथैकस्मिन्नेव दृढे सिद्धे सिद्धासने सति ।
बन्धत्रयमनायासात् स्वयमेवोपजायते ॥४२॥

tathaikasminneva dṛḍhe siddhe siddhāsane sati |
bandhatrayamanāyāsāt svayamevopajāyate ||42||

1.42: When siddhāsana is completely mastered, the three bandha-s follow without any effort.

नासनं सिद्धसदृशं न कुम्भः केवलोपमः ।
न खेचरीसमा मुद्रा न नादसदृशो लयः ॥४३॥

nāsanaṁ siddhasadṛśaṁ na kumbhaḥ kevalopamaḥ |
na khecarīsamā mudrā na nādasadṛśo layaḥ ||43||

1.43: There is no āsana that can equal siddhāsana, no prāṇāyāma like spontaneous stillness of the breath (kevala-kumbhaka), no mudrā like the khecarī (refer chapters III and IV), and no other means of absorption of mind (laya) like that of inner sound or vibration (nāda).

[Krishnamacharya] The khecarī mudrā mentioned here is the one in the fourth chapter, not that from the third chapter.

अथ पद्मासनम् ।
वामोरूपरि दक्षिणं च चरणं संस्थाप्य वामं तथा
दक्षोरूपरि पश्चिमेन विधिना धृत्वा कराभ्यां दृढम् ।
अङ्गुष्ठौ हृदये निधाय चिबुकं नासाग्रमालोकयेदेतद्
व्याधिविनाशकारि यमिनां पद्मासनं प्रोच्यते ॥४४॥

atha padmāsanam |
vāmorūpari dakṣiṇaṁ ca caraṇaṁ saṁsthāpya vāmaṁ tathā dakṣorūpari paścimena vidhinā dhṛtvā karābhyāṁ dṛḍham |
aṅguṣṭhau hṛdaye nidhāya cibukaṁ nāsāgramālokayedetad vyādhivināśakāri yamināṁ padmāsanaṁ procyate ||44||

Now padmāsana [is described].

1.44: Placing the right foot on the left thigh and the left foot on the right thigh, cross the hands behind the back and firmly hold the big toes (the right toe with the right hand and the left toe with the left hand). Place the chin on the chest and gaze at the tip of the nose. This is called padmāsana and it destroys the diseases in those with self-restraint.

[Krishnamacharya] The centers in the navel, heart, and crown of the head are kept in good function by padmāsana, shoulderstand, and headstand respectively. Hence these three are important āsana-s for health.

उत्तानौ चरणौ कृत्वा ऊरुसंस्थौ प्रयत्नतः ।
ऊरुमध्ये तथोत्तानौ पाणी कृत्वा ततो दृशौ ॥४५॥

uttānau caraṇau kṛtvā ūrusaṁsthau prayatnataḥ |
ūrumadhye tathottānau pāṇī kṛtvā tato dṛśau ||45||

नासाग्रे विन्यसेद् राजदन्तमूले तु जिह्वया।
उत्तम्भ्य चिबुकं वक्षस्युत्थाप्य पवनं शनैः॥४६॥

nāsāgre vinyased rājadantamūle tu jihvayā |
uttambhya cibukaṁ vakṣasyutthāpya pavanaṁ śanaiḥ ||46||

1.45-46: Another view (about padmāsana): Place both feet, soles up, on the opposite thighs. Place both the hands, palms facing upwards, on the respective thighs. Gaze at the tip of the nose and place the tip of the tongue at the root of the front teeth. Place the chin on the chest and slowly draw the prāṇa upwards (through mūla-bandha).

[Krishnamacharya] This version of padmāsana includes jālandhara-bandha and mūla-bandha.

इदं पद्मासनं प्रोक्तं सर्वव्याधिविनाशनम् ।
दुर्लभं येन केनापि धीमता लभ्यते भुवि ॥४७॥

idaṁ padmāsanaṁ proktaṁ sarvavyādhivināśanam |
durlabhaṁ yena kenāpi dhīmatā labhyate bhuvi ||47||

1.47: This is called padmāsana which destroys all diseases. It is hard to be attained by most people; only the wise can attain it.

कृत्वा सम्पुटितौ करौ दृढतरं बद्ध्वा तु पद्मासनं
गाढं वक्षसि सन्निधाय चिबुकं ध्यायंश्च तच्चेतसि ।
वारंवारमपानमूर्ध्वमनिलं प्रोत्सारयन् पूरितं
न्यञ्चन् प्राणमुपैति बोधमतुलं शक्तिप्रभावान्नरः ॥४८॥

kṛtvā samputitau karau dṛḍhataraṁ baddhvātu padmāsanaṁ
gāḍhaṁ vakṣasi sannidhāya cibukaṁ dhyāyaṁśca taccetasi |
vāraṁvāramapānamūrdhvamanilaṁ protsārayan pūritaṁ
nyañcan prāṇamupaiti bodhamatulaṁ śaktiprabhāvānnaraḥ ||48||

1.48: Assuming padmāsana well, with the palms facing upwards placed one on top of the other, place the chin firmly on the chest. Meditating on brahman, repeatedly draw the apāna upwards and bring the prāṇa downwards. By this one attains unequalled insight through the power of kuṇḍalinī.

[Krishnamacharya] This is a description of prāṇāyāma with the bandhās and meditation on the Divine in padmāsana.

पद्मासने स्थितो योगी नाडीद्वारेण पूरितम् ।
मारुतं धारयेद्यस्तु स मुक्तो नात्र संशयः ॥४९॥

padmāsane sthito yogī nāḍīdvāreṇa pūritam |
mārutaṁ dhārayedyastu sa mukto nātra saṁśayaḥ ||49||

1.49: The yogi, seated in padmāsana, by steadying the breath drawn in through the nāḍī-s, attains freedom. There is no doubt about this.

[Krishnamacharya] By freedom, the text means that the yogi is less disturbed by the distractions of the world outside. While siddhāsana is more for monks, padmāsana is more for householders. If classical padmāsana is not possible, do it with one leg crossed over the other, or just sit cross-legged.

अथ सिंहासनम् ।
गुल्फौ च वृषणस्याधः सीवन्याः पार्श्वयोः क्षिपेत् ।
दक्षिणे सव्यगुल्फं तु दक्षगुल्फं तु सव्यके ॥५०॥

atha siṁhāsanam |
gulphau ca vṛṣaṇasyādhaḥ sīvanyāḥ pārśvayoḥ kṣipet |
dakṣiṇe savyagulphaṁ tu dakṣagulphaṁ tu savyake ||50||

Now simhāsana [is described].

1.50: Place the ankles on either side of the perineum, the right ankle on the left side, and the left ankle on the right side.

हस्तौ तु जान्वोः संस्थाप्य स्वाङ्गुलीः सम्प्रसार्य च ।
व्यात्तवक्त्रो निरीक्षेत नासाग्रं सुसमाहितः ॥५१॥

hastau tu jānvoḥ saṁsthāpya svāṅgulīḥ samprasārya ca |
vyāttavaktro nirīkṣeta nāsāgraṁ susamāhitaḥ ||51||

1.51: Placing the hands on the knees, spread the fingers and with the mouth wide open [and tongue extended,] gaze at the tip of the nose with a concentrated mind.

सिंहासनं भवेदेतत् पूजितं योगिपुङ्गवैः ।
बन्धत्रितयसन्धानं कुरुते चासनोत्तमम् ॥५२॥

siṁhāsanaṁ bhavedetatpūjitaṁ yogipuṅgavaiḥ |
bandhatritayasandhānaṁ kurute cāsanottamam ||52||

1.52: This is simhāsana, held in high esteem by the great yogis. This excellent āsana facilitates the three bandha-s.

अथ भद्रासनम् ।
गुल्फौ च वृषणस्याधः सीवन्याः पार्श्वयोः क्षिपेत् ।
सव्यगुल्फं तथा सव्ये दक्षगुल्फं तु दक्षिणे ॥५३॥

atha bhadrāsanam |
gulphau ca vṛṣaṇasyādhaḥ sīvanyāḥ pārśvayoḥ kṣipet |
savyagulphaṁ tathā savye dakṣagulphaṁ tu dakṣiṇe ||53||

Now bhadrāsana [is described].

1.53: Place the ankles below the generative organ at the sides of the perineum, the left ankle on the left side, and the right ankle on the right side.

पार्श्वपादौ च पाणिभ्यां दृढं बद्ध्वा सुनिश्चलम् ।
भद्रासनं भवेदेतत् सर्वव्याधिविनाशनम् ।
गोरक्षासनमित्याहुरिदं वै सिद्धयोगिनः ॥५४॥

pārśvapādau ca pāṇibhyāṁ dṛḍhaṁ baddhvā suniścalam |
bhadrāsanaṁ bhavedetat sarvavyādhivināśanam |
gorakṣāsanamityāhuridaṁ vai siddhayoginaḥ ||54||

1.54: Then hold the feet which are on their sides, firmly with the hands and remain without movement. This is bhadrāsana which destroys all diseases. The yogis and adepts (siddha-s) call this gorakṣāsana.

31/01/76: This bhadrāsana is also called gorakṣāsana by the siddha-s.

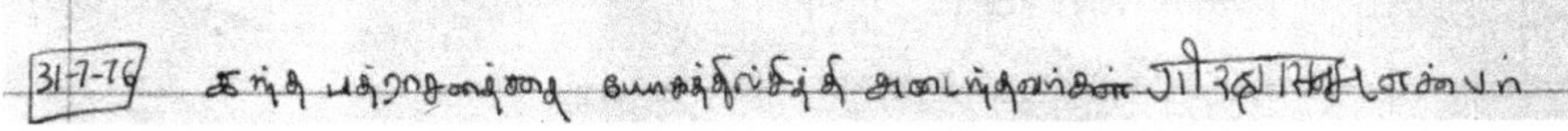

[Krishnamacharya] This can be considered advanced baddha-koṇāsana. The feet are drawn in under the perineum. This āsana is not ideal for women.

एवमासनबन्धेषु योगीन्द्रो विगतश्रमः ।
अभ्यसेन्नाडिकाशुद्धिं मुद्रादिपवनक्रियाम् ॥५५॥

evamāsanabandheṣu yogīndro vigataśramaḥ |
abhyasennāḍikāśuddhiṁ mudrādipavanakriyām ||55||

1.55: Thus, the best of the yogis, when the practice of āsana-s and bandha-s become effortless, should practice cleansing of the nāḍī-s, mudrā-s etc., and control the breath.

आसनं कुम्भकं चित्रं मुद्राख्यं करणं तथा ।
अथ नादानुसन्धानमभ्यासानुक्रमो हठे ॥५६॥

āsanaṁ kumbhakaṁ citraṁ mudrākhyaṁ karaṇaṁ tathā |
atha nādānusandhānamabhyāsānukramo haṭhe ||56||

1.56: Āsana-s, various kinds of prāṇāyāma (kumbhaka), the practices called mudrā, then nādānusandhāna, comprise the sequence of practice in haṭha-yoga.

[Krishnamacharya] This verse list the four parts of the practice which are each described in one chapter in this book.

The following section describes the foods acceptable to a yogi.

ब्रह्मचारी मिताहारी त्यागी योगपरायणः।
अब्दादूर्ध्वं भवेत्सिद्धो नात्र कार्या विचारणा॥५७॥

brahmacārī mitāhārī tyāgī yogaparāyaṇaḥ |
abdādūrdhvaṁ bhavetsiddho nātra kāryā vicāraṇā ||57||

1.57: The celibate (brahmacārī, one who follows sexual restraint) who follows a moderate diet, who is non-attached, and intent on yoga, attains success within a year. There need not be any doubt about this.

सुस्निग्धमधुराहारश्चतुर्थांशविवर्जितः ।
भुज्यते शिवसंप्रीत्यै मिताहारः स उच्यते ॥५८॥

susnigdhamadhurāhāraścaturthāṁśavivarjitaḥ |
bhujyate śivasaṁprītyai mitāhāraḥ sa ucyate ||58||

1.58: Moderate diet (mita-āhāra) means moist and sweet food. It should be eaten as an offering to please Śiva, leaving one-fourth of the stomach empty.

[Krishnamacharya] The purpose of moist food (milk, ghee) is that the practices of bandha-s and prāṇāyāma can result in dryness in the intestinal tract. Hence this is a balance to it.

कट्वम्लतीक्ष्णलवणोष्णहारितशाकसौवीरतैलतिलसर्षपमद्यमत्स्यान्।
आजादिमांसदधितक्रकुलत्थकोलपिण्याकहिङ्गुलशुनाद्यमपथ्यमाहुः॥५९॥

kaṭvamlatīkṣṇalavaṇoṣṇahāritaśākasauvīratailatilasarṣapamadyamatsyān |
ājādimāṁsadadhitakrakulatthakolapiṇyākahiṅgulaśunādyamapathyamāhuḥ ||59||

1.59: The following are said to be unsalutary [for yogis]: foods that are bitter, sour, pungent, salty, heating, radish and vegetables other than those prescribed, sour gruel, [sesame and mustard] oils, sesame, mustard, alcohol, fish, meat including that of the goat, curds, buttermilk, horse-gram, the fruit of the jujube, oil cakes, asafoetida, and garlic.

भोजनमहितं विद्यात् पुनरस्योष्णीकृतं रूक्षम् ।
अतिलवणमम्लयुक्तं कदशनशाकोत्कटं वर्ज्यम् ॥ ६० ॥

bhojanamahitaṁ vidyāt punarasyoṣṇīkṛtaṁ rūkṣam |
atilavaṇamamlayuktaṁ kadaśanaśākotkaṭaṁ varjyam ||60||

1.60: The following should be avoided as unhealthy: food that is reheated, dry foods, foods that have excess salt or sourness, and vegetables [other than those prescribed].

वह्निस्त्रीपथिसेवानामादौ वर्जनमाचरेत् ।
तथा हि गोरक्षवचनम्—
वर्जयेद् दुर्जनप्रान्तं वह्निस्त्रीपथिसेवनम् ।
प्रातःस्नानोपवासादि कायक्लेशविधिं तथा ॥ ६१ ॥

vahnistrīpathisevānāmādau varjanamācaret |
tathā hi gorakṣavacanam–

varjayed durjanaprāntaṁ vahnistrīpathisevanam |
prātaḥsnānopavāsādi kāyakleśavidhiṁ tathā ||61||

1.61: In the beginning, indulgence in fire, women, and long journeys should be avoided. In this regard Gorakṣa says, "Association with bad company, fire, women, and long journeys, bathing early in the morning, fasting, and strenuous physical activity should be avoided."

गोधूमशालियवषाष्टिकशोभनान्नं क्षीराज्यखण्डनवनीतसितामधूनि ।
शुण्ठीपटोलकफलादिकपञ्चशाकं मुद्गादि दिव्यमुदकं च यमीन्द्रपथ्यम् ॥ ६२ ॥

godhūmaśāliyavaṣāṣṭikaśobhanānnaṁ kṣīrājyakhaṇḍanavanītasitāmadhūni |
śuṇṭhīpaṭolakaphalādikapañcaśākaṁ mudgādi divyamudakaṁ ca yamīndrapathyam ||62||

1.62: The following food items are suitable to be taken by the yogi: wheat, rice, barley, the grain called ṣaṣṭika, purified food, milk, ghee, brown sugar, butter, sugar-candy, honey, dry ginger, vegetables such as patola (a variety of cucumber) and the five pot-herbs, green gram, and pure water.

पुष्टं सुमधुरं स्निग्धं गव्यं धातुप्रपोषणम् ।
मनोऽभिलषितं योग्यं योगी भोजनमाचरेत्॥ ६३ ॥

puṣṭaṁ sumadhuraṁ snigdhaṁ gavyaṁ dhātuprapoṣaṇam |
mano'bhilaṣitaṁ yogyaṁ yogī bhojanamācaret ||63||

1.63: The yogi should take sweet food mixed with ghee and milk which is nourishing. It should nourish the tissues and be pleasing and suitable.

Importance of practice for success:

युवा वृद्धोऽतिवृद्धो वा व्याधितो दुर्बलोऽपि वा ।
अभ्यासात् सिद्धिमाप्नोति सर्वयोगेष्वतन्द्रितः ॥ ६४ ॥

yuvā vṛddho'tivṛddho vā vyādhito durbalo'pi vā |
abhyāsāt siddhimāpnoti sarvayogeṣvatandritaḥ ||64||

1.64: Anyone who is not lazy in the pursuit of yoga, whether young, old, very old, ill, or weak, attains success through practice.

[Krishnamacharya] Naturally, the practice is to be designed according to the capacity and needs of the individual. (This was a key principle in Krishnamacharya's teachings.)

क्रियायुक्तस्य सिद्धिः स्यादक्रियस्य कथं भवेत् ।
न शास्त्रपाठमात्रेण योगसिद्धिः प्रजायते ॥ ६५ ॥

kriyāyuktasya siddhiḥ syādakriyasya kathaṁ bhavet |
na śāstrapāṭhamātreṇa yogasiddhiḥ prajāyate ||65||

1.65: One who is intent on practice will attain success. How can anyone who is lazy be successful? Success in yoga is not attained by merely studying the texts (śāstra-s).

[Krishnamacharya] The commentary points out that success is attained not just by practice but only by practicing all the eight limbs of yoga.

न वेषधारणं सिद्धेः कारणं न च तत्कथा ।
क्रियैव कारणं सिद्धेः सत्यमेतन्न संशयः ॥ ६६ ॥

na veṣadhāraṇaṁ siddheḥ kāraṇaṁ na ca tatkathā |
kriyaiva kāraṇaṁ siddheḥ satyametanna saṁśayaḥ ||66||

1.66: Success is not attained by wearing the clothes [of a yogi] or by talking about it. Practice alone is the cause of success. This is the truth without any doubt.

पीठानि कुम्भकाश्चित्रा दिव्यानि करणानि च।
सर्वाण्यपि हठाभ्यासे राजयोगफलावधि॥ ६७॥

pīṭhāni kumbhakāścitrā divyāni karaṇāni ca|
sarvāṇyapi haṭhābhyāse rājayogaphalāvadhi||67||

1.67: The āsana-s, the different kinds of prāṇāyāma (kumbhaka-s), and the excellent mudrā-s of haṭha-yoga should be practiced till the fruit of rāja-yoga is attained.

Chapter II

Chapter II: Detailed Summary

1: Prāṇāyāma: when to start.

2-3: Why practice prāṇāyāma? Breath and mind relationship.

4: Samādhi (nāda) is not possible unless impurities in the nāḍī-s are removed.

5: Why is nāḍī cleansing prāṇāyāma described first?

6: How long should one do prāṇāyāma everyday with a sattva dominant mind?

7-9: Nāḍīśodhana prāṇāyāma.

10: How long does purification of the nāḍī-s (nāḍīśuddhi) take?

11: How many prāṇāyāma-s to practice each day?

12-13: The three stages of prāṇāyāma and their progress.

14: Food guidelines.

15-16: Cautions in doing prāṇāyāma-s.

17: Impairment in the flow of prāṇa results in diseases.

18: The need to regulate the breath gradually.

19: Signs of purification of the nāḍī-s.

20: Benefits of nāḍīśodhana.

21: Who should practice the kriyā-s?

22: List of six kriyā-s.

23: Kriyā-s are to be practiced in privacy.

24: Dhauti—description and methodology.

25: Benefits of dhauti.

26: Vasti—description and methodology.

27-28: Benefits of vasti.

29: Neti—description and methodology.

30: Benefits of neti.

31: Trāṭaka—description and methodology.

32: Benefits of trāṭaka.

33: Nauli—description and methodology.

34: Benefits of nauli.

35: Kapālabhāti—description and methodology.

36: Practice prāṇāyāma after kriyā-s.

37: No need for kriyās; prāṇāyāma is sufficient.

38: Gajakaraṇī.

39: Importance of the practice of prāṇāyāma.

40: Prāṇāyāma and steadiness of mind.

41: Prāṇa enters suṣumnā effortlessly.

42: Prāṇa entering suṣumnā makes mind steady.

43: Practice of prāṇāyāma and siddhi-s.

44: Eight types of prāṇāyāma.

45: Bandha-s.

46: Through proper practice of jālandhara-bandha, uḍḍīyāna-bandha, and mūla-bandha, prāṇa enters suṣumnā.

47: Proper practice gives energy to perform actions.

48-49: Sūryabhedana prāṇāyāma.

50: Benefits of sūryabhedana prāṇāyāma.

51: Ujjāyī prāṇāyāma.

52-53: Benefits of ujjāyī prāṇāyāma.

54: Śītkārī prāṇāyāma.

55: Benefits of śītkārī prāṇāyāma.

56: Sattva arises from the practice.

57: Śītalī prāṇāyāma.

58: Benefits of śītalī prāṇāyāma.

59: Bhastrikā prāṇāyāma.

60: Padmāsana.

61-64: Cautions of bhastrikā prāṇāyāma.

65: Benefits of bhastrikā prāṇāyāma.

66: Prāṇāyāma and the doṣa-s.

67: Bhastrikā prāṇāyāma loosens the three knots.

68: Bhrāmarī prāṇāyāma.

69: Mūrcchā prāṇāyāma.

70: Plāvinī prāṇāyāma.

71-72: Kevala-kumbhaka.

75: Attainment of rāja-yoga.

76-77: There is no rāja-yoga without haṭha-yoga.

78: Experienced results of haṭha-yoga.

Chapter II: Translation

अथासने दृढे योगी वशी हितमिताशनः ।
गुरूपदिष्टमार्गेण प्राणायामान् समभ्यसेत् ॥१॥

athāsane dṛḍhe yogī vaśī hitamitāśanaḥ |
gurūpadiṣṭamārgeṇa prāṇāyāmān samabhyaset ||1||

II.1: The yogi, having become competent in the practice of the āsana-s, with his senses under control, and following an appropriate and moderate diet, should practice prāṇāyāma, according to the instructions of his guru.

[Krishnamacharya] From the seated postures suggested, choose one. The phrase "athāsane" used here is similar to the introduction to Yoga Sūtra II.49 on prāṇāyāma (tasmin sati śvāsapraśvāsayoḥ gati viccedaḥ prāṇāyāmaḥ).

चले वाते चलं चित्तं निश्चले निश्चलं भवेत् ।
योगी स्थाणुत्वमाप्नोति ततो वायुं निरोधयेत् ॥२॥

cale vāte calaṁ cittaṁ niścale niścalaṁ bhavet |
yogī sthāṇutvamāpnoti tato vāyuṁ nirodhayet ||2||

II.2: When the breath is disturbed, the mind is unsteady. When the breath becomes focused, the mind becomes focused, and the yogi attains steadiness. Therefore, the breath should be restrained.

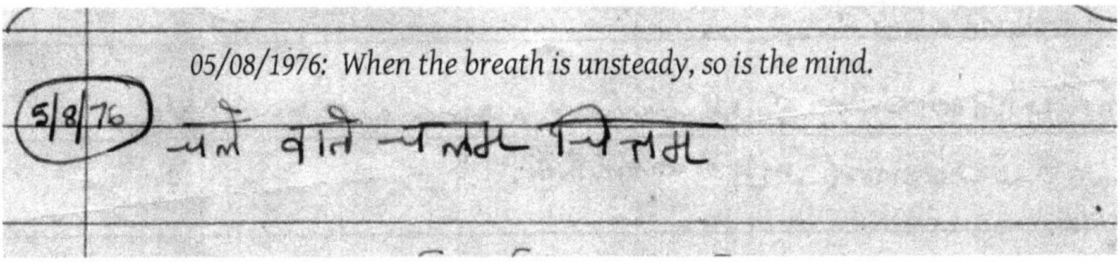
05/08/1976: When the breath is unsteady, so is the mind.

5/8/76 चले वाते चलम् चित्तम्

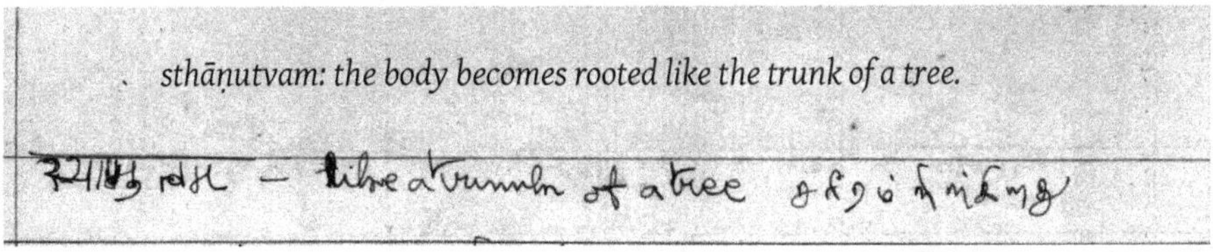
sthāṇutvam: the body becomes rooted like the trunk of a tree.

स्थाणुत्वम् – like a trunk of a tree

[Krishnamacharya] Both suspension after exhalation and holding after inhalation should be practiced to control the prāṇa.

यावद्वायुः स्थितो देहे तावज्जीवनमुच्यते ।
मरणं तस्य निष्क्रान्तिस्ततो वायुं निरोधयेत् ॥ ३ ॥

yāvadvāyuḥ sthito dehe tāvajjīvanamucyate |
maraṇaṁ tasya niṣkrāntistato vāyuṁ nirodhayet ||3||

II.3: Life exists so long as breath (prāṇa) remains in the body. When prāṇa leaves the body, it is death. Therefore, one should restrain the breath.

[Krishnamacharya] Not practicing prāṇāyāma leads to more disease and mental unsteadiness, which in turn reduce life span.

मलाकुलासु नाडीषु मारुतो नैव मध्यगः ।
कथं स्यादुन्मनीभावः कार्यसिद्धिः कथं भवेत् ॥ ४ ॥

malākulāsu nāḍīṣu māruto naiva madhyagaḥ |
kathaṁ syādunmanībhāvaḥ kāryasiddhiḥ kathaṁ bhavet ||4||

II.4: When the nāḍī-s are full of impurities, the breath does not flow into the center (the central nāḍī or suṣumnā). How can one then attain the unmanī-avasthā (state of absorption or samādhi)? How can the goal be attained?

शुद्धिमेति यदा सर्वं नाडीचक्रं मलाकुलम् ।
तदैव जायते योगी प्राणसङ्ग्रहणे क्षमः ॥ ५ ॥

śuddhimeti yadā sarvaṁ nāḍīcakraṁ malākulam |
tadaiva jāyate yogī prāṇasaṅgrahaṇe kṣamaḥ ||5||

II.5: When all the nāḍī-s are purified, only then will the yogi will be able to control his breath (prāṇa).

[Krishnamacharya] The word saṅgraha refers to withdrawal of the sensations caused by prāṇa. Refer Yoga Yājñavalkya, which says that prāṇa is reduced from 108 to 96 aṅgula-s (a unit of measurement).

Only when the nāḍī-s becomes clear does the yogi becomes fit to attain samādhi.

प्राणायामं ततः कुर्यान्नित्यं सात्त्विकया धिया ।
यथा सुषुम्नानाडीस्था मलाः शुद्धिं प्रयान्ति च ॥६॥

prāṇāyāmaṁ tataḥ kuryānnityaṁ sāttvikayā dhiyā |
yathā suṣumnānāḍīsthā malāḥ śuddhiṁ prayānti ca ||6||

II.6: Therefore, prāṇāyāma should be practiced every day with a pure (sāttvika) mind so that the suṣumnā nāḍī is cleansed.

[Krishnamacharya] In the Yoga Yājñavalkya, the whole of Chapter V is dedicated to nāḍīśodhana prāṇāyāma.

Nāḍīśodhana prāṇāyāma is not a cleansing technique (kriyā). The kriyā-s suggested subsequently in this text are external and gross. As the name suggests, nāḍīśodhana prāṇāyāma can cleanse all the nāḍī-s, and therefore, sages such as Yājñavalkya say that prāṇāyāma is itself sufficient and the kriyā-s are unnecessary.

Prāṇāyāma should be done till one attains insight into and experience of the nābhi-cakra referred to in Yoga Sūtra III.29.

बद्धपद्मासनो योगी प्राणं चन्द्रेण पूरयेत् ।
धारयित्वा यथाशक्ति भूयः सूर्येण रेचयेत् ॥७॥

baddhapadmāsano yogī prāṇaṁ candreṇa pūrayet |
dhārayitvā yathāśakti bhūyaḥ sūryeṇa recayet ||7||

II.7: The yogi, seated in padmāsana, should inhale through the left nostril (moon, iḍā nāḍī). He should retain it as long as possible and then exhale through the right nostril (sun, piṅgalā nāḍī).

प्राणं सूर्येण चाकृष्य पूरयेदुदरं शनैः ।
विधिवत्कुम्भकं कृत्वा पुनश्चन्द्रेण रेचयेत् ॥८॥

prāṇaṁ sūryeṇa cākṛṣya pūrayedudaraṁ śanaiḥ |
vidhivatkumbhakaṁ kṛtvā punaścandreṇa recayet ||8||

II.8: [Again] inhaling slowly through the right nostril (sun, piṅgalā nāḍī) and filling the interior, practice kumbhaka (retention) and then exhale through the left nostril (moon, iḍā nāḍī).

येन त्यजेत्तेन पीत्वा धारयेदतिरोधतः ।
रेचयेच्च ततोऽन्येन शनैरेव न वेगतः ॥९॥

yena tyajettena pītvā dhārayedatirodhataḥ |
recayecca tato'nyena śanaireva na vegataḥ ||9||

II.9: Inhaling through the same [nostril] through which the exhalation was done, retain the breath to the extent possible, and exhale through the other [nostril] slowly.

[Krishnamacharya] Never exhale fast. Exhale should always be long, subtle, and smooth. Exhaling fast makes a person lose power and control. Use a mantra to measure the duration of the practice of prāṇāyāma.

प्राणं चेदिडया पिबेन्नियमितं भूयोऽन्यया रेचयेत्
पीत्वा पिङ्गलया समीरणमथो बद्ध्वा त्यजेद् वामया ।
सूर्याचन्द्रमसोरनेन विधिनाभ्यासं सदा तन्वतां
शुद्धा नाडिगणा भवन्ति यमिनां मासत्रयादूर्ध्वतः ॥१०॥

prāṇaṁ cediḍayā pibenniyamitaṁ bhūyo'nyayā recayet
pītvā piṅgalayā samīraṇamatho baddhvā tyajed vāmayā |
sūryācandramasoranena vidhinābhyāsaṁ sadā tanvatāṁ
śuddhā nāḍigaṇā bhavanti yamināṁ māsatrayādūrdhvataḥ ||10||

II.10: If prāṇa is drawn in through the left nostril (moon, iḍā nāḍī), it should be exhaled through the other (right) [nostril] (sun, piṅgalā nāḍī) after retention. If inhaled through the right nostril it should be retained and exhaled through the left [nostril]. In those who follow the yama-s and who practice like this, all the nāḍī-s are purified after three months.

[Krishnamacharya] The practice of prāṇāyāma will lead to cleansing of the nāḍī-s only if accompanied by a moderate and sattva dominant diet.

प्रातर्मध्यन्दिने सायमर्धरात्रे च कुम्भकान् ।
शनैरशीतिपर्यन्तं चतुर्वारं समभ्यसेत् ॥११॥

prātarmadhyandine sāyamardharātre ca kumbhakān |
śanairaśītiparyantaṁ caturvāraṁ samabhyaset ||11||

II.11: One should practice retention (kumbhaka-s) four times a day, in the early morning, at noon, in the evening, and at midnight, gradually until a count of eighty is reached.

[Krishnamacharya] Practice at least three times a day. Do at least twenty-four prāṇāyāma-s twice a day. As you grow older, increase it to thirty prāṇāyāma-s per session.

Krishnamacharya used to tell me do at least 108 slow and deep breaths a day, for good health, inclusive of the number of breaths practiced in āsana.

कनीयसि भवेत् स्वेदः कम्पो भवति मध्यमे ।
उत्तमे स्थानमाप्नोति ततो वायुं निबन्धयेत् ॥१२॥

kanīyasi bhavet svedaḥ kampo bhavati madhyame |
uttame sthānamāpnoti tato vāyuṁ nibandhayet ||12||

II.12: At the lowest stage, there is sweating; at the middle stage, there is trembling; and at the highest stage, the body becomes rooted to earth like a tree. Therefore, one should control the breath.

[Krishnamacharya] Here is a more useful explanation based on practice, which may be a little different from the author as well as the commentator.

In the middle stage, the body does not tremble. The body tries to rise because of the holding in of the breath. The restricted breath tries to expand outward, and hence there is a feeling as if the body wants to lift off the ground. This is called frog-like movement (maṇḍūka-pluti).

During this middle stage of the practice, one should restrain this tendency of the body to rise, and keep the body firm. This is firm āsana (dṛḍha-āsana)—refer ghaṭa-avasthā in IV.72 for correlation.

In the highest stage, the feeling is that the body becomes firm and motionless like a rock. The yogi feels one with the earth and the body sensation is transcended. This is called sthāṇu (refer II.2 above).

The commentator explains the concept of udghāta which is mentioned in the commentaries on Yoga Sūtra II.50 as well. Udghāta refers to the process of performing a certain number of cycles of breathing with a specified length of holding after inhalation and/or suspension after exhalation. For example, it could be 12 cycles of breathing, with 12 seconds of holding after inhalation and/or 12 seconds of suspension after exhalation.

The key here is that the breath should not be forced. This is the implication of the word "udghāta" which literally means "to strike upwards." There should be no feeling of gasping or difficulty in breathing in this practice—the breath should not "strike upwards."

Depending on the duration of the suspension, the practice of udghāta is classified in three stages of advancement. The particular length of breathing in each stage varies in the descriptions of different authors.

जलेन श्रमजातेन गात्रमर्दनमाचरेत् ।
दृढता लघुता चैव तेन गात्रस्य जायते ॥१३॥

jalena śramajātena gātramardanamācaret |
dṛḍhatā laghutā caiva tena gātrasya jāyate ||13||

II.13: Perspiration resulting from the prāṇāyāma should be rubbed on the body. By this massage the body becomes strong and light.

[Krishnamacharya] The yogi used to practice bare-chested, alone in a cave. The principle behind rubbing perspiration into the body is to maintain or conserve the heat (agni) in the body.

अभ्यासकाले प्रथमे शस्तं क्षीराज्यभोजनम् ।
ततोऽभ्यासे दृढीभूते न तादृङ्नियमग्रहः ॥१४॥

abhyāsakāle prathame śastaṁ kṣīrājyabhojanam |
tato'bhyāse dṛḍhībhūte na tādṛṅniyamagrahaḥ ||14||

II.14: In the early stages of the practice, food that contains milk and ghee is prescribed. Once the practice becomes advanced (i.e. stable), such restrictions need not be observed.

[Krishnamacharya] Milk and ghee are suggested in the initial stages to reduce the increased internal heat caused by the increased metabolism (agni). The practice of three bandha-s with prāṇāyāma enhances the metabolism.

Advancement in the practice is inferred when a person can control the breath cycle up to a length of three minutes. There should be no shortness of breath in the practice.

Food restrictions "need not be observed," means that the person should take more solid, sattva-dominant food. Some foods such as chillies must still be avoided.

यथा सिंहो गजो व्याघ्रो भवेद् वश्यः शनैः शनैः ।
तथैव सेवितो वायुरन्यथा हन्ति साधकम् ॥ १५ ॥

yathā siṁho gajo vyāghro bhaved vaśyaḥ śanaiḥ śanaiḥ |
tathaiva sevito vāyuranyathā hanti sādhakam ||15||

II.15: Just as a lion, elephant, or tiger is tamed gradually, the breath too should be brought under control [slowly]. Else it will kill the practitioner.

[Krishnamacharya] If the breath is forced, it will result in chest pain and other heart ailments.

प्राणायामेन युक्तेन सर्वरोगक्षयो भवेत् ।
अयुक्ताभ्यासयोगेन सर्वरोगसमुद्भवः ॥ १६ ॥

prāṇāyāmena yuktena sarvarogakṣayo bhavet |
ayuktābhyāsayogena sarvarogasamudbhavaḥ ||16||

II.16: Through the proper practice of prāṇāyāma [along with proper diet and bandha-s] there is freedom from all diseases. Improper practice of yoga (i.e. prāṇāyāma) results in the manifestation of all diseases.

हिक्का श्वासश्च कासश्च शिरःकर्णाक्षिवेदनाः ।
भवन्ति विविधा रोगाः पवनस्य प्रकोपतः ॥ १७ ॥

hikkā śvāsaśca kāsaśca śiraḥkarṇākṣivedanāḥ |
bhavanti vividhā rogāḥ pavanasya prakopataḥ ||17||

II.17: Hiccups, asthma, bronchial diseases, ear ache, pain in the eyes, and various other diseases can manifest through the wrong practice of prāṇāyāma.

[Krishnamacharya] Impairment in the flow of prāṇa results in many diseases.

युक्तं युक्तं त्यजेद् वायुं युक्तं युक्तं च पूरयेत् ।
युक्तं युक्तं च बध्नीयादेवं सिद्धिमवाप्नुयात् ॥ १८ ॥

yuktaṁ yuktaṁ tyajed vāyuṁ yuktaṁ yuktaṁ ca pūrayet |
yuktaṁ yuktaṁ ca badhnīyādevaṁ siddhimavāpnuyāt ||18||

II.18: One should exhale appropriately (slowly and attentively) and inhale appropriately (slowly and attentively). Then, one should appropriately (comfortably and attentively) restrain the breath. Only then will the benefits of the practice be attained.

[Krishnamacharya] Holding the breath after inhalation and suspension after exhalation should be introduced and practiced gradually.

यदा तु नाडीशुद्धिः स्यात् तथा चिह्नानि बाह्यतः ।
कायस्य कृशता कान्तिस्तदा जायेत निश्चितम् ॥ १९ ॥

yadā tu nāḍīśuddhiḥ syāt tathā cihnāni bāhyataḥ |
kāyasya kṛśatā kāntistadā jāyeta niścitam ||19||

II.19: When the nāḍī-s are purified, external signs arise, such as leanness of the body accompanied by radiance, certainly.

[Krishnamacharya] The yogi should always be lean.

यथेष्टं धारणं वायोरनलस्य प्रदीपनम् ।
नादाभिव्यक्तिरारोग्यं जायते नाडिशोधनात् ॥ २० ॥

yatheṣṭaṁ dhāraṇaṁ vāyoranalasya pradīpanam |
nādābhivyaktirārogyaṁ jāyate nāḍiśodhanāt ||20|

II.20: When the nāḍī-s are purified, one is capable of restraining the breath as desired, the metabolism (agni) is stimulated, the inner sound (nāda) is heard, and there is good health.

[Krishnamacharya] All the above benefits accrue through the practice of nāḍīśodhana prāṇāyāma itself.

मेदश्लेष्माधिकः पूर्वं षट्कर्माणि समाचरेत् ।
अन्यस्तु नाचरेत्तानि दोषणां समभावतः ॥ २१ ॥

medaśleṣmādhikaḥ pūrvaṁ ṣaṭkarmāṇi samācaret |
anyastu nācarettāni doṣaṇāṁ samabhāvataḥ ||21||

II.21: One who is overweight and has excess phlegm, should first (before the practice of prāṇāyāma) practice the six acts (cleansing techniques or kriyā-s).

Others [who do not have these issues] should not practice them, because the three doṣa-s (vāta, pitta, and kapha) are balanced in them.

[Krishnamacharya] Six kriyā-s are described in Haṭha Yoga Pradīpikā. These six kriyā-s are divided into further categories in the Gheraṇḍa Samhitā.

These kriyā-s are not related to kriyā-yoga in Yoga Sutra II.1.

Some of the kriyā-s involve using solids (e.g. a piece of cloth) and liquids (e.g. water). The distance between the lower cakra-s is potentially disturbed by these practices. Moreover, some of these practices may also directly disturb the nervous system.

The practice of gazing (trāṭaka) is useful and can be an aid to meditation.

The fast breathing technique (kapālabhāti) is useful if practiced in limited cycles, appropriately.

The practice of nauli can be done, sometimes, but only with proper prāṇāyāma practice and the bandha-s.

In young practitioners, the kriyā-s may not cause health disturbances and the body may recover quickly from their impact, whereas in older persons, it could aggravate the underlying health issues. (Though Krishnamacharya demonstrated nauli, he did not normally teach it to students.)

The Haṭha Yoga Pradīpikā is a later text. The more ancient yogi-s did not speak about the uses of kriyā-s. Control over diet, with proper practice of āsana and prāṇāyāma, should usually be sufficient to keep the doṣa-s in balance. If the doṣa-s are out of balance, Ayurveda or other health measures may be needed rather than the kriyā-s.

धौतिर्बस्तिस्तथा नेतिस्त्राटकं नौलिकं तथा ।
कपालभातिश्चैतानि षट्कर्माणि प्रचक्षते ॥२२॥

dhautirbastistathā netistrāṭakaṁ naulikaṁ tathā |
kapālabhātiścaitāni ṣaṭkarmāṇi pracakṣate ||22||

II.22: The six acts (cleansing techniques or kriyā-s) are dhauti, vasti, neti, trāṭaka, nauli, and kapālabhāti.

कर्मषट्कमिदं गोप्यं घटशोधनकारकम् ।
विचित्रगुणसन्धायि पूज्यते योगिपुङ्गवैः ॥२३॥

karmaṣaṭkamidaṁ gopyaṁ ghaṭaśodhanakārakam |
vicitraguṇasandhāyi pūjyate yogipuṅgavaiḥ ||23||

II.23: These six acts (cleansing techniques or kriyā-s), which purify the body and produce special benefits, should be kept secret. They are held in high esteem by great yogis.

तत्र धौतिः ।
चतुरङ्गुलविस्तारं हस्तपञ्चदशायतम् ।
गुरूपदिष्टमार्गेण सिक्तं वस्त्रं शनैर्ग्रसेत् ।
पुनः प्रत्याहरेच्चैतदुदितं धौतिकर्म तत् ॥२४॥

tatra dhautiḥ |
caturaṅgulavistāraṁ hastapañcadaśāyatam |
gurūpadiṣṭamārgeṇa siktaṁ vastraṁ śanairgraset |
punaḥ pratyāhareccaitaduditaṁ dhautikarma tat ||24||

Now dhauti [is described].

II.24: Slowly swallow a wet piece of cloth, four aṅgula-s (i.e. four finger widths) broad and fifteen spans long, as instructed by the guru. Then draw it out. This process is called dhauti.

कासश्वासप्लीहकुष्ठं कफरोगाश्च विंशतिः ।
धौतिकर्मप्रभावेण प्रयान्त्येव न संशयः ॥२५॥

kāsaśvāsaplīhakuṣṭhaṁ kapharogāśca viṁśatiḥ |
dhautikarmaprabhāveṇa prayāntyeva na saṁśayaḥ ||25||

II.25: By the efficacy of dhauti, cough, asthma, diseases of the spleen (plīha), skin disorders, and twenty other diseases brought on by excess kapha disappear. This is beyond doubt.

अथ बस्तिः ।
नाभिदघ्नजले पायौ न्यस्तनालोत्कटासनः ।
आधाराकुञ्चनं कुर्यात् क्षालनं बस्तिकर्म तत् ॥२६॥

atha bastiḥ |
nābhidaghnajale pāyau nyastanālotkaṭāsanaḥ |
ādhārākuñcanaṁ kuryāt kṣālanaṁ bastikarma tat ||26||

Now vasti [is described].

II.26: Squatting (i.e. utkaṭāsana) in water up to the navel, insert a [small bamboo] tube into the anus and contract the anus [so as to draw the water in and then expel it]. Such cleansing is called vasti.

गुल्मप्लीहोदरं चापि वातपित्तकफोद्भवाः ।
बस्तिकर्मप्रभावेण क्षीयन्ते सकलामयाः ॥२७॥

gulmaplīhodaraṁ cāpi vātapittakaphodbhavāḥ |
bastikarmaprabhāveṇa kṣīyante sakalāmayāḥ ||27||

II.27: By the efficacy of vasti, tumours, diseases of the spleen (plīha), dropsy and other stomach disorders, and all diseases [arising from imbalance of doṣa-s] are cured.

धात्विन्द्रियान्तःकरणप्रसादं दद्याच्च कान्तिं दहनप्रदीप्तिम् ।
अशेषदोषोपचयं निहन्यादभ्यस्यमानं जलबस्तिकर्म ॥२८॥

dhātvindriyāntaḥkaraṇaprasādaṁ dadyācca kāntiṁ dahanapradīptim |
aśeṣadoṣopacayaṁ nihanyādabhyasyamānaṁ jalabastikarma ||28||

II.28: This vasti with water, when practiced [properly], refines the tissues (dhatu-s), the senses (indriya-s) and the mind (antaḥkarana). It gives luster to the body and increases the digestive power. It destroys all accumulation of doṣa-s in the body.

अथ नेतिः ।
सूत्रं वितस्ति सुस्निग्धं नासानाले प्रवेशयेत् ।
मुखान्निर्गमयेच्चैषा नेतिः सिद्धैर्निगद्यते ॥२९॥

atha netiḥ |
sūtraṁ vitasti susnigdhaṁ nāsānāle praveśayet |
mukhānnirgamayeccaiṣā netiḥ siddhairnigadyate ||29||

Now neti [is described].

II.29: Insert a smooth thread [about nine inches long] through the nasal passage and draw it out through the mouth. The adepts (siddha-s) call this neti.

कपालशोधिनी चैव दिव्यदृष्टिप्रदायिनी ।
जत्रूर्ध्वजातरोगौघं नेतिराशु निहन्ति च ॥३०॥

kapālaśodhinī caiva divyadṛṣṭipradāyinī |
jatrūrdhvajātarogaughaṁ netirāśu nihanti ca ||30||

II.30: Neti purifies the skull and enables one to perceive subtle things. Neti also removes all diseases of the body above the shoulders.

अथ त्राटकम् ।
निरीक्षेन्निश्चलदृशा सूक्ष्मलक्ष्यं समाहितः ।
अश्रुसम्पातपर्यन्तमाचार्यैस्त्राटकं स्मृतम् ॥३१॥

atha trāṭakam |
nirīkṣenniścaladṛśā sūkṣmalakṣyaṁ samāhitaḥ |
aśrusampātaparyantamācāryaistrāṭakaṁ smṛtam ||31||

Now trāṭaka [is described].

II.31: Gaze [without blinking] at a minute object, with concentration, until tears are shed. This is called trāṭaka by the ācārya-s (guru-s).

मोचनं नेत्ररोगाणां तन्द्रादीनां कपाटकम् ।
यत्नतस्त्राटकं गोप्यं यथा हाटकपेटकम् ॥३२॥

mocanaṁ netrarogāṇāṁ tandrādīnāṁ kapāṭakam |
yatnatastrāṭakaṁ gopyaṁ yathā hāṭakapeṭakam ||32||

II.32: Trāṭaka removes all diseases of the eye, dullness etc. It should be kept secret and carefully guarded like a casket of gold.

अथ नौलिः ।
अमन्दावर्तवेगेन तुन्दं सव्यापसव्यतः ।
नतांसो भ्रामयेदेषा नौलिः सिद्धैः प्रशस्यते ॥३३॥

atha naulih |
amandāvartavegena tundaṁ savyāpasavyataḥ |
natāṁso bhrāmayedeṣā nauliḥ siddhaiḥ praśasyate ||33||

Now nauli [is described].

II.33: With the shoulders bent forward, the abdomen should be rotated swiftly to right and left. This is called nauli by the adepts (siddha-s).

मन्दाग्निसन्दीपनपाचनादिसन्धापिकानन्दकरी सदैव ।
अशेषदोषामयशोषणी च हठक्रियामौलिरियं च नौलिः ॥३४॥

mandāgnisandīpanapācanādisandhāpikānandakarī sadaiva |
aśeṣadoṣāmayaśoṣaṇī ca haṭhakriyāmauliriyaṁ ca nauliḥ ||34||

II.34: Nauli, the crown of haṭha-yoga practice, stimulates the metabolism (agni) when it is dull, thereby increasing the digestive power, brings about happiness, and destroys all diseases and disorders of the doṣa-s.

अथ कपालभातिः ।
भस्त्रावल्लोहकारस्य रेचपूरौ ससंभ्रमौ ।
कपालभातिर्विख्याता कफदोषविशोषणी ॥३५॥

atha kapālabhātiḥ |
bhastrāvallohakārasya recapūrau sasaṁbhramau |
kapālabhātirvikhyātā kaphadoṣaviśoṣaṇī ||35||

Now kapālabhāti [is described].

II.35: Inhaling and exhaling rapidly like the bellows of a blacksmith is called kapālabhāti. It destroys all diseases caused by kapha.

षट्कर्मनिर्गतस्थौल्यकफदोषमलादिकः ।
प्राणायामं ततः कुर्यादनायासेन सिध्यति ॥३६॥

ṣaṭkarmanirgatasthaulyakaphadoṣamalādikaḥ |
prāṇāyāmaṁ tataḥ kuryādanāyāsena siddhyati ||36||

II.36: Freed from excess weight, kapha disorders etc. through the practice of the six acts (cleansing techniques or kriyā-s), one should practice prāṇāyāma. Then success is attained without much strain.

प्राणायामैरेव सर्वे प्रशुष्यन्ति मला इति ।
आचार्याणां तु केषाञ्चिदन्यत्कर्म न संमतम् ॥ ३७ ॥

prāṇāyāmaireva sarve praśuṣyanti malā iti |
ācāryāṇāṁ tu keṣāñcidanyatkarma na saṁmatam ||37||

II.37: Some teachers do not accept the kriyā-s since they consider that all the impurities in the system are removed by the practice of prāṇāyāma alone.

[Krishnamacharya] The commentator mentions that the acārya-s like Yājñavalkya do not approve of the practice of these cleansing techniques.

अथ गजकरणी ।
उदरगतपदार्थमुद्वमन्ति पवनमपानमुदीर्य कण्ठनाले ।
क्रमपरिचयवश्यनाडिचक्रा गजकरणीति निगद्यते हठज्ञैः ॥ ३८ ॥

atha gajakaraṇī |
udaragatapadārthamudvamanti pavanamapānamudīrya kaṇṭhanāle |
kramaparicayavaśyanāḍicakrā gajakaraṇīti nigadyate haṭhajñaiḥ ||38||

Now gajakaraṇī [is described].

II.38: Drawing up the apāna to the throat, vomit the substances (i.e. food and water) that are in the stomach. This practice which gradually brings all nāḍī-s under control is called gajakaraṇī by practitioners of haṭha-yoga.

[Krishnamacharya] Gajakaraṇī is mentioned between the kriyā-s and the prāṇāyāma techniques that follow. Gajakaraṇī is a result (siddhi) based on bandha-s and not a kriyā. It does not involve any external aids unlike other kriyā-s.

ब्रह्मादयोऽपि त्रिदशाः पवनाभ्यासतत्पराः ।
अभूवन्नन्तकभयात् तस्मात् पवनमभ्यसेत् ॥ ३९ ॥

brahmādayo'pi tridaśāḥ pavanābhyāsatatparāḥ |
abhūvannantakabhayāt tasmāt pavanamabhyaset ||39||

II.39: Even Brahmā and other gods devoted themselves to the practice of prāṇāyāma because of the fear of death. Therefore, one should practice control of breath.

Important: Practice prāṇāyāma whenever you can find the time!

[Krishnamacharya] Practice prāṇāyāma whenever you get time.

यावद् बद्धो मरुद् देहे यावच्चित्तं निराकुलम् ।
यावद् दृष्टिर्भ्रुवोर्मध्ये तावत् कालभयं कुतः ॥४०॥

yāvad baddho marud dehe yāvaccittaṁ nirākulam |
yāvad dṛṣṭirbhruvormadhye tāvat kālabhayaṁ kutaḥ ||40||

II.40: As long as breath (prāṇa) is retained in the body through prāṇāyāma, as long as the mind is in a state of balance, and as long as the gaze is directed to the center of the eyebrows, why should one fear death?

विधिवत् प्राणसंयामैर्नाडीचक्रे विशोधिते ।
सुषुम्नावदनं भित्त्वा सुखाद् विशति मारुतः ॥४१॥

vidhivat prāṇasaṁyāmairnāḍīcakre viśodhite |
suṣumnāvadanaṁ bhittvā sukhādviśati mārutaḥ ||41||

II.41: When the nāḍī-s are purified through the proper practice of prāṇāyāma, the breath (prāṇa) opens the mouth of suṣumnā and easily enters it.

अथ मनोन्मनी ।
मारुते मध्यसञ्चारे मनःस्थैर्यं प्रजायते ।
यो मनःसुस्थिरीभावः सैवावस्था मनोन्मनी ॥४२॥

atha manonmanī |
mārute madhyasañcāre manaḥsthairyaṁ prajāyate |
yo manaḥsusthirībhāvaḥ saivāvasthā manonmanī ||42||

Now manonmanī [is described].

II.42 When the prāṇa flows through the suṣumnā, the mind becomes steady. This steadiness of the mind is called manonmanī.

[Krishnamacharya] By nāḍīśodhana prāṇāyāma, the scattered mind becomes centered or focused. This is very useful for meditation. Steadiness of the body is attained through āsana practice. Steadiness of the mind is attained through prāṇāyāma.

तत्सिद्धये विधानज्ञाश्चित्रान्कुर्वन्ति कुम्भकान् ।
विचित्रकुम्भकाभ्यासाद् विचित्रां सिद्धिमाप्नुयात् ॥४३॥

tatsiddhaye vidhānajñāścitrānkurvanti kumbhakān |
vicitrakumbhakābhyāsād vicitrāṁ siddhimāpnuyāt ||43||

II.43: To attain that state of absorption (unmanī or samādhi), learned practitioners practice various types of kumbhaka-s (prāṇāyāma-s). Through the practice of various types of kumbhaka-s, diverse special results (siddhi-s) are obtained.

अथ कुम्भकभेदाः ।
सूर्यभेदनमुज्जायी सीत्कारी शीतली तथा ।
भस्त्रिका भ्रामरी मूर्च्छा प्लाविनीत्यष्ट कुम्भकाः ॥४४॥

atha kumbhakabhedāḥ |
sūryabhedanamujjāyī sītkārī śītalī tathā |
bhastrikā bhrāmarī mūrcchā plāvinītyaṣṭa kumbhakāḥ ||44||

Now the different kumbhaka-s [are described]:

II.44: There are eight kumbhaka-s, namely sūryabhedana, ujjāyī, sītkārī, śītalī, bhastrikā, bhrāmarī, mūrcchā, and plāvinī.

पूरकान्ते तु कर्तव्यो बन्धो जालन्धरभिधः ।
कुम्भकान्ते रेचकादौ कर्तव्यस्तूड्डीयानकः ॥४५॥

pūrakānte tu kartavyo bandho jalandharabhidhaḥ |
kumbhakānte recakādau kartavyastūḍḍīyānakaḥ ||45||

II.45: Jālandhara-bandha is practiced (maintained) at the end of inhalation. At the end of kumbhaka and at the beginning of exhalation, uḍḍīyāna-bandha must be practiced.

[Krishnamacharya] Jālandhara-bandha should be practiced in postures before introducing it in prāṇāyāma.

अधस्तात् कुञ्चनेनाशु कण्ठसङ्कोचने कृते ।
मध्ये पश्चिमतानेन स्यात् प्राणो ब्रह्मनाडिगः ॥४६॥

adhastāt kuñcanenāśu kaṇṭhasaṅkocane kṛte |
madhye paścimatānena syāt prāṇo brahmanāḍigaḥ ||46||

II.46: Contract the throat [with jālandhara-bandha] and draw the perineum upwards [with mūla-bandha] at the same time, and then contract the abdomen [with uḍḍīyāna-bandha]. Then the prāṇa flows through the suṣumnā (brahmanāḍī).

अपानमूर्ध्वमुत्थाप्य प्राणं कण्ठादधो नयेत् ।
योगी जराविमुक्तः सन् षोडशाब्दवया भवेत् ॥४७॥

apānamūrdhvamutthāpya prāṇaṁ kaṇṭhādadho nayet |
yogī jarāvimuktaḥ san ṣoḍaśābdavayā bhavet ||47||

II.47: Raising the apāna upwards [with mūla-bandha] the prāṇa should be brought down the throat [with jālandhara-bandha]. Then the yogi becomes youthful like a sixteen-year old, free from old age.

[Krishnamacharya] All the three bandha-s must be learned and mastered in āsana-s with breath control. The text can be misleading. At the highest level, the only bandha to be practiced is uḍḍīyāna-bandha, since jālandhara-bandha and mūla-bandha are supposed to be maintained throughout the practice of prāṇāyāma.

[Mohan] The Haṭha Yoga Pradīpikā describes eight types of prāṇāyāma, but Krishnamacharya taught many more. The descriptions of the practices in these verses miss numerous practical details. In 1979, before I had to do a seminar on prāṇāyāma in Switzerland, Krishnamacharya went into detail on the subject of prāṇāyāma for over six months.

अथ सूर्यभेदनम् ।
आसने सुखदे योगी बद्धा चैवासनं ततः ।
दक्षनाड्या समाकृष्य बहिःस्थं पवनं शनैः ॥४८॥
आकेशादानखाग्राच्च निरोधावधि कुम्भयेत् ।
ततः शनैः सव्यनाड्या रेचयेत् पवनं शनैः ॥४९॥

atha sūryabhedanam |
āsane sukhade yogī baddhvā caivāsanaṁ tataḥ |
dakṣanāḍyā samākṛṣya bahiḥsthaṁ pavanaṁ śanaiḥ ||48||

ākeśādānakhāgrācca nirodhāvadhi kumbhayet |
tataḥ śanaiḥ savyanāḍyā recayet pavanaṁ śanaiḥ ||49||

Now sūryabhedana [is described].

II.48: Assuming the proper posture on a comfortable seat, draw in air through the right nostril (piṅgalā).

II.49: Then, practice kumbhaka, retaining [the breath] till it is felt from the hair [on the head] to the tip of the toe nails (pervading the whole body). Then exhale slowly through the left nostril (iḍā).

कपालशोधनं वातदोषघ्नं कृमिदोषहृत् ।
पुनः पुनरिदं कार्यं सूर्यभेदनमुत्तमम् ॥५०॥

kapālaśodhanaṁ vātadoṣaghnaṁ kṛmidoṣahṛt |
punaḥ punaridaṁ kāryaṁ sūryabhedanamuttamam ||50||

II.50: This sūryabhedana, which is the best, should be repeatedly practiced, as it purifies the head, cures diseases arising from vāta, and maladies caused by worms.

अथोज्जायी ।
मुखं संयम्य नाडीभ्यामाकृष्य पवनं शनैः ।
यथा लगति कण्ठात्तु हृदयावधि सस्वनम् ॥५१॥
पूर्ववत् कुम्भयेत् प्राणं रेचयेदिडया तथा ।

athojjāyī |
mukhaṁ saṁyamya nāḍībhyāmākṛṣya pavanaṁ śanaiḥ |
yathā lagati kaṇṭhāttu hṛdayāvadhi sasvanam ||51||
pūrvavat kumbhayet prāṇaṁ recayediḍayā tathā |

Now ujjāyī [is described].

II.51: Closing the mouth, inhale slowly through both nostrils from the throat to the heart [feeling a rubbing sensation in the throat].

II.52: Then practice kumbhaka as previously [instructed in sūryabhedana] and exhale the breath through the left nostril (iḍā).

[Krishnamacharya] During inhalation, the feeling should be from the neck till the diaphragm. Alternate nostril exhalation is to be inferred.

श्लेष्मदोषहरं कण्ठे देहानलविवर्धनम् ॥५२॥
नाडीजलोदराधातुगतदोषविनाशनम् ।
गच्छता तिष्ठता कार्यमुज्जाय्याख्यं तु कुम्भकम् ॥५३॥

śleṣmadoṣaharaṁ kaṇṭhe dehānalavivardhanam ||52||
nāḍījalodarādhātugatadoṣavināśanam |
gacchatā tiṣṭhatā kāryamujjāyyākhyaṁ tu kumbhakam ||53||

II.52: This removes disorders in the throat caused by kapha and kindles the metabolism in the body.

II.53: It also put an end to diseases in the nāḍī-s, tissues (dhātu-s), and dropsy. This kumbhaka known as ujjāyī can be practiced while walking or standing.

अथ सीत्कारी–
सीत्कां कुर्यात्तथा वक्त्रे घ्राणेनैव विजृम्भिकाम् ।
एवमभ्यासयोगेन कामदेवो द्वितीयकः ॥५४॥

atha sītkārī–
sītkāṁ kuryāttathā vaktre ghrāṇenaiva vijṛmbhikām |
evamabhyāsayogena kāmadevo dvitīyakaḥ ||54||

Now sītkārī [is described].

II.54: Make a hissing sound with the mouth [while inhaling] and exhale only through the nostrils. By repeated practice in this way, one becomes like a second god of beauty (kāma-deva).

योगिनीचक्रसंमान्यः सृष्टिसंहारकारकः ।
न क्षुधा न तृषा निद्रा नैवालस्यं प्रजायते ॥५५॥

yoginīcakrasaṁmānyaḥ sṛṣṭisaṁhārakārakaḥ |
na kṣudhā na tṛṣā nidrā naivālasyaṁ prajāyate ||55||

II.55: He (i.e. the yogi who practices sītkārī) is highly regarded among yogini-s. He is always energetic. Hunger, thirst, sleep and indolence do not arise in him.

भवेत्सत्त्वं च देहस्य सर्वोपद्रववर्जितम् ।
अनेन विधिना सत्यं योगीन्द्रो भूमिमण्डले ॥५६॥

bhavetsattvaṁ ca dehasya sarvopadravavarjitam |
anena vidhinā satyaṁ yogīndro bhūmimaṇḍale ||56||

II.56: By this practice bodily strength is increased and the best among yogi-s truly becomes free from all afflictions in this world.

अथ शीतली–
जिह्वया वायुमाकृष्य पूर्ववत् कुम्भसाधनम् ।
शनकैर्घ्राणरन्ध्राभ्यां रेचयेत् पवनं सुधीः ॥५७॥

atha śītalī–
jihvayā vāyumākṛṣya pūrvavat kumbhasādhanam |
śanakairghrāṇarandhrābhyāṁ recayet pavanaṁ sudhīḥ ||57||

Now śītalī [is described].

II.57: Curling the tongue [and protruding it a little outside the lips], inhale and hold the breath as before. Then exhale slowly through the nostrils.

गुल्मप्लीहादिकान् रोगान् ज्वरं पित्तं क्षुधां तृषाम् ।
विषाणि शीतली नाम कुम्भिकेयं निहन्ति हि ॥५८॥

gulmaplīhādikān rogān jvaraṁ pittaṁ kṣudhāṁ tṛṣām |
viṣāṇi śītalī nāma kumbhikeyaṁ nihanti hi ||58||

II.58: This kumbhaka named śītalī destroys diseases of the abdomen, spleen etc., and also fever, pitta related diseases, hunger, thirst, and [the bad effects of] poisons.

अथ भस्त्रिका–
ऊर्वोरुपरि संस्थाप्य शुभे पादतले उभे ।
पद्मासनं भवेदेतत् सर्वपापप्रणाशनम् ॥५९॥
सम्यक् पद्मासनं बद्ध्वा समग्रीवोदरः सुधीः ।
मुखं संयम्य यत्नेन प्राणं घ्राणेन रेचयेत् ॥६०॥
यथा लगति हृत्कण्ठे कपालावधि सस्वनम् ।
वेगेन पूरयेच्चापि हृत्पद्मावधि मारुतम् ॥६१॥

atha bhastrikā–
ūrvorupari saṁsthāpya śubhe pādatale ubhe |
padmāsanaṁ bhavedetat sarvapāpapraṇāśanam ||59||

samyak padmāsanaṁ baddhvā samagrīvodaraḥ sudhīḥ |
mukhaṁ saṁyamya yatnena prāṇaṁ ghrāṇena recayet ||60||

yathā lagati hṛtkaṇṭhe kapālāvadhi sasvanam |
vegena pūrayeccāpi hṛtpadmāvadhi mārutam ||61||

Now bhastrikā [is described].

II.59-61: When both feet are placed on the opposite thighs, it is called padmāsana, which destroys all ill effects or sins (pāpa). Seated in padmāsana properly, with the neck and the abdomen in line, the wise practitioner should close the mouth and exhale through the nostrils with force until it is felt to resound in the chest, throat, and up to the skull. Then inhale rapidly till it reaches the lotus of the heart.

[Krishnamacharya] In the kapālabhāti prāṇāyāma, the speed (i.e. the number of breaths per minute) is important. In bhastrikā, it is the force with which the air is expelled that is important. Bhastrikā is used for awakening the kuṇḍalinī, involving more effort from the lowest three cakras, whereas kapālabhāti involves more effort from the chest.

पुनर्विरेचयेत् तद्वत् पूरयेच्च पुनः पुनः ।
यथैव लोहकारेण भस्त्रा वेगेन चाल्यते ॥६२॥
तथैव स्वशरीरस्थं चालयेत्पवनं धिया ।
यदा श्रमो भवेद् देहे तदा सूर्येण पूरयेत् ॥६३॥

punarvirecayet tadvat pūrayecca punaḥ punaḥ |
yathaiva lohakāreṇa bhastrā vegena cālyate ||62||

tathaiva svaśarīrasthaṁ cālayetpavanaṁ dhiyā |
yadā śramo bhaved dehe tadā sūryeṇa pūrayet ||63||

II.62-63: Exhale in the same manner and inhale, again and again. Similar to a blacksmith working his bellows with speed, one should mindfully stimulate the prāṇa in the body [by exhalation and inhalation]. When the body feels tired, breathe in through the right nostril.

[Krishnamacharya] If this practice is not interspersed with sufficient inhalation and a little holding after inhalation, dizziness may arise.

यथोदरं भवेत्पूर्णमनिलेन तथा लघु ।
धारयेन्नासिकां मध्यातर्जनीभ्यां विना दृढम् ॥६४॥

yathodaraṁ bhavetpūrṇamanilena tathā laghu |
dhārayennāsikāṁ madhyātarjanībhyāṁ vinā dṛḍham ||64||

II.64: After expanding the abdomen, the nostrils should be closed using the thumb, the ring finger, and the little finger (mṛgī-mudrā).

विधिवत् कुम्भकं कृत्वा रेचयेदिडयानिलम् ।
वातपित्तश्लेष्महरं शरीराग्निविवर्धनम् ॥६५॥

vidhivat kumbhakaṁ kṛtvā recayediḍayānilam |
vātapittaśleṣmaharaṁ śarīrāgnivivardhanam ||65||

II.65: After practicing retention (kumbhaka) as prescribed, the breath should be exhaled through the left nostril. This removes [disorders arising from] imbalance of vāta, pitta, and kapha, and stimulates the metabolism (agni).

कुण्डलीबोधकं क्षिप्रं पवनं सुखदं हितम् ।
ब्रह्मनाडीमुखे संस्थकफाद्यर्गलनाशनम् ॥६६॥

kuṇḍalībodhakaṁ kṣipraṁ pavanaṁ sukhadaṁ hitam |
brahmanāḍīmukhe saṁsthakaphādyargalanāśanam ||66||

II.66: Bhastrikā arouses the kuṇḍalinī quickly and is purifying, pleasant, and beneficial. It removes all obstructions caused by kapha from the mouth of the suṣumnā.

सम्यग्गात्रसमुद्भूतग्रन्थित्रयविभेदकम् ।
विशेषेणैव कर्तव्यं भस्त्राख्यं कुम्भकं त्विदम् ॥६७॥

samyaggātrasamudbhūtagranthitrayavibhedakam |
viśeṣeṇaiva kartavyaṁ bhastrākhyaṁ kumbhakaṁ tvidam ||67||

II.67: This kumbhaka called bhastrikā should be specially practiced since it breaks through the three knots (granthi-s) created in the body.

अथ भ्रामरी–
वेगाद्घोषं पूरकं भृङ्गनादं भृङ्गीनादं रेचकं मन्दमन्दम् ।
योगीन्द्राणामेवमभ्यासयोगाच्चित्ते जाता काचिदानन्दलीला ॥६८॥

atha bhrāmarī–
vegādghoṣaṁ pūrakaṁ bhṛṅganādaṁ bhṛṅgīnādaṁ recakaṁ mandamandam |
yogīndrāṇāmevamabhyāsayogāccitte jātā kācidānandalīlā ||68||

Now bhrāmarī [is described].

II.68: Breathe in rapidly with a sound resembling the humming of a male bee, then exhale slowly [after retention] making the humming sound of a female bee. By this practice, immense bliss is experienced by the best of the yogis.

अथ मूर्च्छा–
पूरकान्ते गाढतरं बद्ध्वा जालन्धरं शनैः ।
रेचयेन्मूर्च्छनाख्येयं मनोमूर्च्छा सुखप्रदा ॥६९॥

atha mūrcchā–
pūrakānte gāḍhataraṁ baddhvā jalandharaṁ śanaiḥ |
recayenmūrcchanākhyeyaṁ manomūrcchā sukhapradā ||69||

Now mūrcchā [is described].

II.69: At the end of inhalation, practicing jālandhara-bandha firmly, exhale slowly. This is called mūrcchā as it reduces the mind to a state of inactivity and bestows happiness.

[Krishnamacharya] This prāṇāyāma with long exhalation is helpful in sleeping disorders.

अथ प्लाविनी–
अन्तःप्रवर्तितोदारमारुतापूरितोदरः ।
पयस्यगाधेऽपि सुखात् प्लवते पद्मपत्रवत् ॥७०॥

atha plāvinī–
antaḥpravartitodāramārutāpūritodaraḥ |
payasyagādhe'pi sukhāt plavate padmapatravat ||70||

Now plāvinī [is described].

II.70: Owing to the interior of the body being abundantly filled by deep inhalation, [the yogi] floats easily like a lotus leaf, even in deep waters.

प्राणायामस्त्रिधा प्रोक्तो रेचपूरककुम्भकैः ।
सहितः केवलश्चेति कुम्भको द्विविधो मतः ॥७१॥

prāṇāyāmastridhā prokto recapūrakakumbhakaiḥ |
sahitaḥ kevalaśceti kumbhako dvividho mataḥ ||71||

II.71: Prāṇāyāma is said to be threefold, exhale (recaka), inhale (pūraka), and holding (kumbhaka). Kumbhaka is of two kinds, sahita and kevala.

यावत् केवलसिद्धिः स्यात् सहितं तावदभ्यसेत् ।
रेचकं पूरकं मुक्त्वा सुखं यद् वायुधारणम् ॥७२॥
प्राणायामोऽयमित्युक्तः स वै केवलकुम्भकः ।
कुम्भके केवले सिद्धे रेचपूरकवर्जिते ॥७३॥

yāvat kevalasiddhiḥ syāt sahitaṁ tāvadabhyaset |
recakaṁ pūrakaṁ muktvā sukhaṁ yad vāyudhāraṇam ||72||
prāṇāyāmo'yamityuktaḥ sa vai kevalakumbhakaḥ |
kumbhake kevale siddhe recapūrakavarjite ||73||

II.72-73: One should practice holding with inhalations and exhalations (sahita-kumbhaka) until kevala-kumbhaka is achieved. When the breath is held with ease without exhalation or inhalation this is called kevala-kumbhaka.

न तस्य दुर्लभं किञ्चित् त्रिषु लोकेषु विद्यते ।
शक्तः केवलकुम्भेन यथेष्टं वायुधारणात् ॥७४॥

na tasya durlabhaṁ kiñcit triṣu lokeṣu vidyate |
śaktaḥ kevalakumbhena yatheṣṭaṁ vāyudhāraṇāt ||74||

II.74: When kevala-kumbhaka is mastered, there is nothing that cannot be attained by him (the yogi) in all the three worlds.

[Krishnamacharya] Refer Yoga Yājñavalkya VI.26-35 for a description of kevala-kumbhaka.

राजयोगपदं चापि लभते नात्र संशयः ।
कुम्भकात् कुण्डलीबोधः कुण्डलीबोधतो भवेत् ।
अनर्गला सुषुम्ना च हठसिद्धिश्च जायते ॥७५॥

rājayogapadaṁ cāpi labhate nātra saṁśayaḥ |
kumbhakāt kuṇḍalībodhaḥ kuṇḍalībodhato bhavet |
anargalā suṣumnā ca haṭhasiddhiśca jāyate ||75||

II.75: Through the mastery of kevala-kumbhaka even rāja-yoga can be attained. There is no doubt about this. Through kevala-kumbhaka, kuṇḍalinī is aroused. When kuṇḍalinī is aroused, suṣumnā is freed from all obstructions, and perfection in haṭha-yoga is attained.

[Krishnamacharya] In the Haṭha Yoga Pradīpikā, it is said that kevala-kumbhaka leads to rāja-yoga. According to the Yoga Sūtra, there is no success in kevala-kumbhaka without meditation.

हठं विना राजयोगो राजयोगं विना हठः ।
न सिध्यति ततो युग्ममानिष्पत्तेः समभ्यसेत् ॥७६॥

haṭhaṁ vinā rājayogo rājayogaṁ vinā haṭhaḥ |
na sidhyati tato yugmamāniṣpatteḥ samabhyaset ||76||

II.76: Without haṭha-yoga, rāja-yoga cannot be achieved, and without rāja-yoga, haṭha-yoga is of no use. Therefore, both should be practiced until perfection [in rāja-yoga] is attained.

[Krishnamacharya] Without the practice of haṭha-yoga to maintain good health and the foundation of the body for further practices, rāja-yoga does not fructify. Similarly, haṭha-yoga is not useful without rāja-yoga—sattva dominant samādhi—as the goal. Therefore, both must be practiced together till samādhi is attained.

कुम्भकप्राणरोधान्ते कुर्याच्चित्तं निराश्रयम् ।
एवमभ्यासयोगेन राजयोगपदं व्रजेत् ॥७७॥

kumbhakaprāṇarodhānte kuryāccittaṁ nirāśrayam |
evamabhyāsayogena rājayogapadaṁ vrajet ||77||

II.77: During retention of breath in kumbhaka, the mind should be clear (i.e. focused). By this practice the state of rāja-yoga is achieved.

वपुः कृशत्वं वदने प्रसन्नता नादस्फुटत्वं नयने सुनिर्मले ।
अरोगता बिन्दुजयोऽग्निदीपनं नाडीविशुद्धिर्हठसिद्धिलक्षणम् ॥७८॥

vapuḥ kṛśatvaṁ vadane prasannatā nādasphuṭatvaṁ nayane sunirmale |
arogatā bindujayo'gnidīpanaṁ nāḍīviśuddhirhaṭhasiddhilakṣaṇam ||78||

II.78: The signs of perfection in haṭha-yoga are: slimness of body, brightness in the face, manifestation of the inner sound (nāda), clear eyes, absence of illness, control over the seminal fluid, stimulation of the metabolism (agni) and purification of the nāḍī-s.

Chapter III

Chapter III: Detailed Summary

The methods and benefits of practice are presented together in many verses.

1-9: Introductory verses about the mudrā-s.

10-15: Mahāmudrā—description and practice.

16-18: Benefits and praise of mahāmudrā.

19-23: Mahāvedha—description and practice.

24-25: Benefits and praise of mahāvedha.

26-28: Mahābandha—description and practice.

29-31: Benefits and praise of mahābandha.

32: Khecarī—definition.

33-37: Practice of khecarī mudrā.

38-40: Benefits and praise of khecarī mudrā.

41: Why the mudrā is called khecarī.

42-46: Benefits and praise of khecarī mudrā.

47-50: Some details in practicing khecarī mudrā, and its benefits.

51-54: Greatness of khecarī mudrā.

55-57: Uḍḍīyāna-bandha—description and practice.

58-60: Benefits and praise of uḍḍīyāna-bandha.

61-63: Mūla-bandha—description and practice.

64: Benefits and praise of mūla-bandha.

65-69: Practice and benefits of mūla-bandha.

70-72: Jālandhara-bandha—description and practice.

73: Benefits and praise of jālandhara-bandha.

73-76: Benefits of practice of the three bandha-s.

77-79: Viparītakaraṇī—description and practice.

80: Benefits and praise of viparītakaraṇī.

81-82: Pacing of practice of viparītakaraṇī, benefits and praise.

83-91: Vajrolī—description, practice, and benefits.

92-95: Amarolī—description, practice, and benefits.

96-103: Sahajolī—description, practice, and benefits.

104-130: Śakti-cālana—description, practice, and benefits.

Chapter III: Translation

Verses 1-9 deal with the following points:

1. Introduction to the concept of kuṇḍalinī.
2. Importance of kuṇḍalinī according to tantra.
3. How the cakra-s are pierced.
4. When the kuṇḍalinī awakens.
5. How the suṣumnā is the royal path for prāṇa.
6. The need to practice the ten mudrā-s.

सशैलवनधात्रीणां यथाधारोऽहिनायकः ।
सर्वेषां योगतन्त्राणां तथाधारो हि कुण्डली ॥१॥

saśailavanadhātrīṇāṁ yathādhāro'hināyakaḥ |
sarveṣāṁ yogatantrāṇāṁ tathādhāro hi kuṇḍalī ||1||

III.1: Just as the Lord of the Serpents (ananta), is the support of the earth with its mountains and forests, so is kuṇḍalinī the support of all yoga practices.

[Krishnamacharya] Ādhāra also means "basis." In the tantra texts, kuṇḍalinī is the basis for the practices proposed. The goal in haṭha-yoga is to burn the kuṇḍalinī; in śākta traditions, it is to awaken the kuṇḍalinī. This point is repeated throughout this chapter. Kuṇḍalinī is the power of our saṁskāra-s. In the presentation of the Yoga Sūtra, it is our saṁskarā-s that need to be burnt. Burning the kuṇḍalinī philosophically refers to the "burnt seed" (dagdha-bīja) state in Vyāsa's commentary on Yoga Sūtra II.4.

सुप्ता गुरुप्रसादेन यदा जागर्ति कुण्डली ।
तदा सर्वाणि पद्मानि भिद्यन्ते ग्रन्थयोऽपि च ॥२॥

suptā guruprasādena yadā jāgarti kuṇḍalī |
tadā sarvāṇi padmāni bhidyante granthayo'pi ca ||2||

III.2: When the sleeping kuṇḍalinī awakens, and rises through the grace of the Guru then all the lotuses and knots (granthi-s) are pierced.

[Krishnamacharya] The three knots (granthi-s) referred to in IV.70-76 are called that of creation (brahma-granthi), support (viṣṇu-granthi), and destruction (rudra-granthi) respectively. The grace of the guru should be taken as the grace of the Divine.

The commentator Brahmānanda mentions that "all the lotuses" here refers to only the lower six cakra-s, not the seventh at the crown of the head. That is because the piercing of the seventh cakra happens only at the time of the yogi's death. You can see this explained in the Yoga Yājñavalkya XII.34. Krishnamacharya used to say that when the seventh cakrā is pierced, the yogi becomes one with the Divine.

"Piercing of the cakra-s" refers to the awareness of the movement of prāṇa within.

प्राणस्य शून्यपदवी तदा राजपथायते ।
तदा चित्तं निरालम्बं तदा कालस्य वञ्चनम् ॥३॥

prāṇasya śūnyapadavī tadā rājapathāyate |
tadā cittaṁ nirālambaṁ tadā kālasya vañcanam ||3||

III.3: Then, suṣumnā becomes the royal path of prāṇa. Then the mind remains free of objects and death is deceived.

[Krishnamacharya] When kuṇḍalinī is burnt, prāṇa goes into suṣumnā. What this means is that the mind turns inwards and focuses on the self (ātman).

"Kālasya vañcanam" is translated as "death is deceived." It means that the fear of death recedes. How does this happen? The practice of prāṇāyāma with the bandha-s leads to the realization that "I am not the body." The instinctive survival fear—abhiniveśa kleśa as described in Yoga Sūtra II.9—is diminished.

सुषुम्ना शून्यपदवी ब्रह्मरन्ध्रं महापथः ।
श्मशानं शाम्भवी मध्यमार्गश्चेत्येकवाचकाः ॥४॥

suṣumnā śūnyapadavī brahmarandhraṁ mahāpathaḥ |
śmaśānaṁ śāmbhavī madhyamārgaścetyekavācakāḥ ||4||

III.4: Suṣumnā, the great void (śūnyapadavī), the entry to Brahman (brahmarandhra), the great path (mahāpatha), the cremation ground (śmaśāna), the power of Lord Śiva (śāmbhavī) and the central path (madhyamārga)—all these refer to the same.

[Krishnamacharya] Headstand is called brahmarandhrāsana. When headstand is practiced as viparītakaraṇī mudrā it becomes the opening to the door of Brahman (i.e. an expanded state of consciousness).

तस्मात् सर्वप्रयत्नेन प्रबोधयितुमीश्वरीम् ।
ब्रह्मद्वारमुखे सुप्तां मुद्राभ्यासं समाचरेत् ॥५॥

tasmāt sarvaprayatnena prabodhayitumīśvarīm |
brahmadvāramukhe suptāṁ mudrābhyāsaṁ samācaret ||5||

III.5: Therefore, making every effort, the [various] mudrā-s should be practiced to awaken the Goddess (kuṇḍalinī) who sleeps at the mouth of suṣumnā.

[Krishnamacharya] Awakening kuṇḍalinī refers to burning out the kuṇḍalinī blocking suṣumnā. This is repeated in various ways in many verses.

महामुद्रा महाबन्धो महावेधश्च खेचरी ।
उड्डीयानं मूलबन्धश्च बन्धो जालन्धराभिधः ॥६॥
करणी विपरीताख्या वज्रोली शक्तिचालनम् ।
इदं हि मुद्रादशकं जरामरणनाशनम् ॥७॥

mahāmudrā mahābandho mahāvedhaśca khecarī |
uḍḍīyānaṁ mūlabandhaśca bandho jālandharābhidhaḥ ||6||

karaṇī viparītākhyā vajrolī śakticālanam |
idaṁ hi mudrādaśakaṁ jarāmaraṇanāśanam ||7||

III.6-7: Mahāmudrā, mahābandha, mahāvedha, khecarī, uḍḍīyāna-bandha, mūla-bandha, jālandhara-bandha, viparītakaraṇī, vajrolī, and śakticālana are the ten mudrā-s. They destroy old age and death.

[Krishnamacharya] "Destroy old age" means the mudrā-s prevent diseases that arise due to old age. "Destroy death" should be understood as overcoming the fear of death.

आदिनाथोदितं दिव्यमष्टैश्वर्यप्रदायकम्
वल्लभं सर्वसिद्धानां दुर्लभं मरुतामपि ॥८॥

ādināthoditaṁ divyamaṣṭaiśvaryapradāyakam |
vallabhaṁ sarvasiddhānāṁ durlabhaṁ marutāmapi ||8||

III.8: These mudrā-s were expounded by Ādinātha (Lord Śiva). They are Divine and bestow the eight special powers (siddhi-s). The practice of the mudrā-s can protect even the siddha-s (i.e. those who have attained special powers through yoga) and are difficult to attain even by the demigods (deva-s).

[Krishnamacharya] They are "Divine," means that they lead to a state of divinity or freedom from suffering (mokṣa). But mudrā-s are not a direct means to such freedom. Through the practice of mudrā-s, when the prāṇa moves into suṣumnā, a steady state of mind is reached. This in turn leads to freedom through progressively deeper meditation. The demigods (deva-s) are said to be in a state of enjoyment (bhoga) always. Only humans can attain freedom through effort and are therefore considered superior to deva-s in this respect.

गोपनीयं प्रयत्नेन यथा रत्नकरण्डकम् ।
कस्यचिन्नैव वक्तव्यं कुलस्त्रीसुरतं यथा ॥९॥

gopanīyaṁ prayatnena yathā ratnakaraṇḍakam |
kasyacinnaiva vaktavyaṁ kulastrīsuratam yathā ||9||

III.9: This [practice of mudrā-s] must be kept secret like a casket of precious gems. It should not be disclosed to anyone, but kept protected like the woman of a good family (kulastrī).

अथ महामुद्रा ।
पादमूलेन वामेन योनिं सम्पीड्य दक्षिणम् ।
प्रसारितं पदं कृत्वा कराभ्यां धारयेद्दृढम् ॥१०॥
कण्ठे बन्धं समारोप्य धारयेद्वायुमूर्ध्वतः ।
यथा दण्डहतः सर्पो दण्डाकारः प्रजायते ॥११॥
ऋज्वीभूता तथा शक्तिः कुण्डली सहसा भवेत् ।
तदा सा मरणावस्था जायते द्विपुटाश्रया ॥१२॥

ततः शनैः शनैरेव रेचयेन्नैव वेगतः ।
इयं खलु महामुद्रा महासिद्धैः प्रदर्शिता ॥ १३ ॥

atha mahāmudrā |
pādamūlena vāmena yoniṁ sampīḍya dakṣiṇam |
prasāritaṁ padaṁ kṛtvā karābhyāṁ dhārayeddṛḍham ||10||

kaṇṭhe bandhaṁ samāropya dhārayedvāyumūrdhvataḥ |
yathā daṇḍahataḥ sarpo daṇḍākāraḥ prajāyate ||11||

ṛjvībhūtā tathā śaktiḥ kuṇḍalī sahasā bhavet |
tadā sā maraṇāvasthā jāyate dvipuṭāśrayā ||12||

tataḥ śanaiḥ śanaireva recayennaiva vegataḥ |
iyaṁ khalu mahāmudrā mahāsiddhaiḥ pradarśitā ||13||

Now mahāmudrā [is described].

III.10: Pressing the perineum with the left heel, stretch the right leg out and hold it firmly with the hands.

III.11-12: Contracting the throat, direct the breath (prāṇa) upwards into the suṣumnā. Just as a coiled serpent when struck by a rod straightens out like a stick, the coiled kuṇḍalinī becomes straight. Then the other two nāḍī-s (iḍā and piṅgalā) become lifeless.

[Krishnamacharya] The implication of the kuṇḍalinī becoming straight when struck is that it is like a snake that is dead. That is, kuṇḍalinī is destroyed.

The prāṇā enters the suṣumnā, leaving the iḍā and piṅgalā.

III.13: Then breathe out very slowly, not with haste. This is mahāmudrā, described by the great adepts.

[Krishnamacharya] considered mahāmudrā the most important of the mudrā-s. He used to say that mahāmudrā as well as the ṣaṇmukhī mudrā should be practiced for physical and mental well-being. He would also recommend adaptations of mahāmudrā for different health conditions. This mudrā is useful for women, to help with reproductive and menstrual issues.

In Krishnamacharya's view, of the ten mudrā-s prescribed in this text, mahāmudrā, viparītakaraṇī mudrā, and the three bandha-s (jalandhara-, uḍḍīyāna-, and mūla-bandha-s) are sufficient to achieve all the goals of classical haṭha-yoga.

Lack of control over the breath on exhalation will lead to loss of focus and power—this is a point mentioned elsewhere in this text as well.

महाक्लेशादयो दोषाः क्षीयन्ते मरणादयः ।
महामुद्रां च तेनैव वदन्ति विबुधोत्तमाः ॥ १४ ॥

mahākleśādayo doṣāḥ kṣīyante maraṇādayaḥ |
mahāmudrāṁ ca tenaiva vadanti vibudhottamāḥ ||14||

III.14: [By the practice of mahāmudrā] all the afflictions (kleśa-s) and associated illnesses and death are vanquished. Therefore, this is called mahāmudrā by the wisest of men.

[Krishnamacharya] Mudrā-s are the indirect cause of these results. When the mind becomes clear and steady through these practices, the kleśa-s will diminish. The text presents indirect causes as direct causes in many verses.

चन्द्राङ्गे तु समभ्यस्य सूर्याङ्गे पुनरभ्यसेत् ।
यावत्तुल्या भवेत्सङ्ख्या ततो मुद्रां विसर्जयेत् ॥ १५ ॥

candrāṅge tu samabhyasya sūryāṅge punarabhyaset |
yāvattulyā bhavetsaṅkhyā tato mudrāṁ visarjayet ||15||

III.15: After practicing well on the left side, it must be practiced on the right side. When the number [of breaths practiced on each side] is equal, the mudrā should be released.

न हि पथ्यमपथ्यं वा रसाः सर्वेऽपि नीरसाः ।
अपि भुक्तं विषं घोरं पीयूषमिव जीर्यति ॥ १६ ॥

na hi pathyamapathyaṁ vā rasāḥ sarve'pi nīrasāḥ |
api bhuktaṁ viṣaṁ ghoraṁ pīyūṣamiva jīryati ||16||

III.16: [For the practitioner of mahāmudrā] there is no healthy or unhealthy diet. All food, insipid or deadly poison, is digested as if it were nectar.

[Krishnamacharya] This should be taken to mean that even heavy or incompatible food will be digested.

क्षयकुष्ठगुदावर्तगुल्माजीर्णपुरोगमाः ।
तस्य दोषाः क्षयं यान्ति महामुद्रां तु योऽभ्यसेत् ॥ १७ ॥

kṣayakuṣṭhagudāvartagulmājīrṇapurogamāḥ |
tasya doṣāḥ kṣayaṁ yānti mahāmudrāṁ tu yo'bhyaset ||17||

III.17: For the one who practices mahāmudrā, various maladies like consumption, leprosy, constipation, abdominal diseases, indigestion etc. are overcome.

कथितेयं महामुद्रा महासिद्धिकरा नृणाम् ।
गोपनीया प्रयत्नेन न देया यस्य कस्यचित् ॥ १८ ॥

kathiteyaṁ mahāmudrā mahāsiddhikarā nṛṇām |
gopanīyā prayatnena na deyā yasya kasyacit ||18||

III.18: Mahāmudrā, which confers great benefits, has thus been described. This should be carefully guarded and not revealed to any and all.

[Krishnamacharya] Ask about the health history of the student before teaching these practices.

अथ महाबन्धः ।
पार्ष्णिं वामस्य पादस्य योनिस्थाने नियोजयेत् ।
वामोरूपरि संस्थाप्य दक्षिणं चरणं तथा ॥ १९ ॥

atha mahābandhaḥ |
pārṣṇiṁ vāmasya pādasya yonisthāne niyojayet |
vāmorūpari saṁsthāpya dakṣiṇaṁ caraṇaṁ tathā ||19||

Now mahābandha [is described].

III.19: Pressing the perineum with the heel of the left foot, place the right foot on the left thigh.

[Krishnamacharya] While the texts say all three mudrā-s (mahāmudrā, mahābandha, mahāvedha) should be done together, the practice of mahāmudrā alone is sufficient. Mahābandha and mahāvedha are not essential. The latter two are often done forcefully and can be substituted with other practices.

पूरयित्वा ततो वायुं हृदये चिबुकं दृढम् ।
निष्पीड्य वायुमाकुञ्च्य मनोमध्ये नियोजयेत् ॥२०॥

pūrayitvā tato vāyuṁ hṛdaye cibukaṁ dṛḍham |
niṣpīḍya vāyumākuñcya manomadhye niyojayet ||20||

III.20: Inhale and press the chin firmly onto the chest [in jālandhara-bandha]. Contract the perineum (i.e. do mūla-bandha) and fix the mind on the central nāḍī (suṣumnā).

धारयित्वा यथाशक्ति रेचयेदनिलं शनैः ।
सव्याङ्गे तु समभ्यस्य दक्षाङ्गे पुनरभ्यसेत् ॥२१॥

dhārayitvā yathāśakti recayedanilaṁ śanaiḥ |
savyāṅge tu samabhyasya dakṣāṅge punarabhyaset ||21||

III.21: Having retained the breath to the extent possible, it should be exhaled slowly. Having practiced well on the left side, then practice on the right side.

मतमत्र तु केषाञ्चित् कण्ठबन्धं विवर्जयेत् ।
राजदन्तस्थजिह्वायां बन्धः शस्तो भवेदिति ॥२२॥

matamatra tu keṣāñcit kaṇṭhabandhaṁ vivarjayet |
rājadantasthajihvāyāṁ bandhaḥ śasto bhavediti ||22||

III.22: Some are of the view that the contraction of the throat (jālandhara-bandha) should be avoided. [In its place,] the contraction effected by the tongue pressing behind the front teeth is preferred.

अयं तु सर्वनाडीनामूर्ध्वं गतिनिरोधकः ।
अयं खलु महाबन्धो महासिद्धिप्रदायकः ॥२३॥

ayaṁ tu sarvanāḍīnāmūrdhvaṁ gatinirodhakaḥ |
ayaṁ khalu mahābandho mahāsiddhipradāyakaḥ ||23||

III.23: This [jivhā-bandha or contraction effected by the tongue, while engaged in mahā-bandha] stops the upward movement [of the prāṇa] through all the nāḍī-s [except suṣumnā]. This mahā-bandha confers great special powers (siddhi-s).

कालपाशमहाबन्धविमोचनविचक्षणः ।
त्रिवेणीसङ्गमं धत्ते केदारं प्रापयेन्मनः ॥२४॥

kālapāśamahābandhavimocanavicakṣaṇaḥ |
triveṇīsaṅgamaṁ dhatte kedāraṁ prāpayenmanaḥ ||24||

III.24: This frees one from the bondage of time. It brings about the union of the three streams [of iḍā, piṅgalā, and suṣumnā]. It leads the mind to kedāra (i.e. the sacred seat of Śiva, the mystic center between the eyebrows).

रूपलावण्यसम्पन्ना यथा स्त्री पुरुषं विना ।
महामुद्रामहाबन्धौ निष्फलौ वेधवर्जितौ ॥२५॥

rūpalāvaṇyasampannā yathā strī puruṣaṁ vinā |
mahāmudrāmahābandhau niṣphalau vedhavarjitau ||25||

III.25: Just as a woman endowed with beauty and charm is unfruitful without a husband, so are mahāmudrā and mahābandha without mahāvedha.

अथ महावेधः ।
महाबन्धस्थितो योगी कृत्वा पूरकमेकधीः ।
वायूनां गतिमावृत्य निभृतं कण्ठमुद्रया ॥२६॥
समहस्तयुगो भूमौ स्फिचौ सन्ताडयेच्छनैः ।
पुटद्वयमतिक्रम्य वायुः स्फुरति मध्यगः ॥२७॥
सोमसूर्याग्निसम्बन्धो जायते चामृताय वै ।
मृतावस्था समुत्पन्ना ततो वायुं विरेचयेत् ॥२८॥

atha mahāvedhaḥ |
mahābandhasthito yogī kṛtvā pūrakamekadhīḥ |
vāyūnāṁ gatimāvṛtya nibhṛtaṁ kaṇṭhamudrayā ||26||

samahastayugo bhūmau sphicau santāḍayecchanaiḥ |
puṭadvayamatikramya vāyuḥ sphurati madhyagaḥ ||27||

somasūryāgnisambandho jāyate cāmṛtāya vai |
mṛtāvasthā samutpannā tato vāyuṁ virecayet ||28||

Now mahāvedha [is described].

III.26: Assuming mahābandha, the yogi should inhale with a focused mind and stop the [upward and downward] movement of the prāṇa, through jālandhara-bandha.

III.27: Placing both palms straight on the ground, strike [the ground] slowly with the buttocks. Then [the prāṇa] leaving the two naḍī-s (iḍā and piṅgalā) penetrates through the central naḍī (suṣumnā).

III.28: Then, the union of [prāṇa in the] moon channel (iḍā), sun channel (piṅgalā), and the fire [channel] (suṣumnā) takes place. This leads to a death-like state. After this one should exhale slowly.

महावेधोऽयमभ्यासान्महासिद्धिप्रदायकः ।
वलीपलितवेपघ्नः सेव्यते साधकोत्तमैः ॥२९॥

mahāvedho'yamabhyāsānmahāsiddhipradāyakaḥ |
valīpalitavepaghnaḥ sevyate sādhakottamaiḥ ||29||

III.29: This is mahāvedha, which with practice bestows great special powers (siddhi-s). It removes wrinkles, grey hair, and tremors. The best of practitioners devote themselves to this.

एतत्त्रयं महागुह्यं जरामृत्युविनाशनम् ।
वह्निवृद्धिकरं चैव ह्यणिमादिगुणप्रदम् ॥३०॥

etattrayaṁ mahāguhyaṁ jarāmṛtyuvināśanam |
vahnivṛddhikaraṁ caiva hyaṇimādiguṇapradam ||30||

III.30: These three [mudrā-s—mahāmudrā, mahābandha, and mahāvedha—] that ward off old age and death, kindle the metabolism and also bestow special powers such as aṇimā, must be most carefully kept secret.

अष्टधा क्रियते चैव यामे यामे दिने दिने ।
पुण्यसम्भारसन्धायि पापौघभिदुरं सदा ।
सम्यक्शिक्षावतामेवं स्वल्पं प्रथमसाधनम् ॥३१॥

aṣṭadhā kriyate caiva yāme yāme dine dine |
puṇyasambhārasandhāyi pāpaughabhiduraṁ sadā |
samyakśikṣāvatāmevaṁ svalpaṁ prathamasādhanam ||31||

III.31: These are to be done eight times, every day at every three-hour interval (yāma). They always bestow much virtue (puṇya) and destroy the accumulation of sins (pāpa). Those who are well guided [by the teacher] must practice them gradually.

[Krishnamacharya] If practiced eight times every three hours, the count will add up to 64 times a day. This is not practical. After my usual āsana and prāṇāyāma practice, this is what I used to do:

Headstand and shoulderstand for a total of 15 minutes.

Mahāmudrā 12 breaths on each side, for 10-15 minutes. Note the long breath implied by this duration.

This part of the practice, lasting around about 25 minutes, was to be done 3 times a day—in the morning, afternoon, and evening.

अथ खेचरी ।
कपालकुहरे जिह्वा प्रविष्टा विपरीतगा ।
भ्रुवोरन्तर्गता दृष्टिर्मुद्रा भवति खेचरी ॥३२॥

atha khecarī |
kapālakuhare jihvā praviṣṭā viparītagā |
bhruvorantargatā dṛṣṭirmudrā bhavati khecarī ||32||

Now khecarī [is described].

III.32: When the tongue is curled back inward and enters the cavity leading to the skull, and the gaze is fixed between the eyebrows, this is khecarī-mudrā.

[Krishnamacharya] There are two khecarī mudrā-s presented in this text. The first is here in III.32-54 and the second is in IV.43-47.

Krishnamacharya used to label the first as tāntric. The second involves prāṇāyāma, and he used to call it Vedic. His view was that, to attain the benefits of the practice of khecarī mudrā described in Chapter III, the practice of the prāṇāyāma presented in Chapter IV is essential.

Tāntric khecarī in Chapter III involves the tongue entering the kaphāla-kuhara (curling back and upward against the palate and behind). Vedic khecarī in Chapter IV involves prāṇa (breath and awareness) entering that space.

The Vedic khecarī mudrā leads to what is called lambikā-yoga. This is mentioned in the Taittirīya Upaniṣat.

Tāntric khecarī mudrā can result in temporary suppression of the bodily feeling of "I." Vedic khecarī forms a better platform for deeper meditation and is more effective in removing the latent impressions or saṁskāra-s. The Vedic khecarī mudrā is useful in attaining the kevala-kumbhaka state described in the Yoga Sūtra II.51.

The practice of Vedic khecarī also involves the use of bandha-s. Krishnamacharya detailed the methodology during my studies of Chapter IV with him.

छेदनचालनदोहैः कलां क्रमेणाथ वर्धयेत्तावत् ।
सा यावद्भ्रूमध्यं स्पृशति तदा खेचरीसिद्धिः ॥३३॥

chedanacālanadohaiḥ kalāṁ krameṇātha vardhayettāvat |
sā yāvadbhrūmadhyaṁ spṛśati tadā khecarīsiddhiḥ ||33||

III.33: By cutting, wiggling, and stretching it, the tongue should be gradually elongated till it touches the spot between the eyebrows. Then khecarī is successfully accomplished.

स्नुहीपत्रनिभं शस्त्रं सुतीक्ष्णं स्निग्धनिर्मलम् ।
समादाय ततस्तेन रोममात्रं समुच्छिनेत् ॥३४॥

snuhīpatranibhaṁ śastraṁ sutīkṣṇaṁ snigdhanirmalam |
samādāya tatastena romamātraṁ samucchinet ||34||

III.34: Taking a smooth, clean knife which is very sharp like the leaf of the milk hedge plant (snuhi-patra), carefully cut by a hair's breadth [the frenulum or the tender membrane beneath the tongue that connects the tongue to the lower part of the mouth].

ततः सैन्धवपथ्याभ्यां चूर्णिताभ्यां प्रघर्षयेत् ।
पुनः सप्तदिने प्राप्ते रोममात्रं समुच्छिनेत् ॥३५॥

tataḥ saindhavapathyābhyāṁ cūrṇitābhyāṁ pragharṣayet |
punaḥ saptadine prāpte romamātraṁ samucchinet ||35||

III.35: Then rub [the cut surface] with [a compound of] powdered rock salt and chebulic myrobalan (harītakī). After seven days, cut again to the extent of a hair's breadth.

एवं क्रमेण षण्मासं नित्यं युक्तः समाचरेत् ।
षण्मासाद्रसनामूलसिराबन्धः प्रणश्यति ॥३६॥

evaṁ krameṇa ṣaṇmāsaṁ nityaṁ yuktaḥ samācaret |
ṣaṇmāsādrasanāmūlasirābandhaḥ praṇaśyati ||36||

III.36: This should be practiced gradually and skillfully for six months. In six months, the binding membrane at the root of the tongue is severed.

[Krishnamacharya] If the root of the tongue is cut like this, clarity of pronunciation may be affected. This can be a problem when doing chanting, for instance.

कलां पराङ्मुखी कृत्वा त्रिपथे परियोजयेत् ।
सा भवेत्खेचरी मुद्रा व्योमचक्रं तदुच्यते ॥३७॥

kalāṁ parāṅmukhī kṛtvā tripathe pariyojayet |
sā bhavetkhecarī mudrā vyomacakraṁ taducyate ||37||

III.37: Then curling the tongue backwards, it should be made to enter the junction of the three nāḍī-s. This is called khecarī mudrā. It is [also] called vyoma-cakra ("space cakra").

[Krishnamacharya] This is referred to as brahmaguhā-cakra as well. If you wish to have results from doing this type of khecarī, you must practice the khecarī described in Chapter IV.

रसनामूर्ध्वगां कृत्वा क्षणार्धमपि तिष्ठति ।
विषैर्विमुच्यते योगी व्याधिमृत्युजरादिभिः ॥३८॥

rasanāmūrdhvagāṁ kṛtvā kṣaṇārdhamapi tiṣṭhati |
viṣairvimucyate yogī vyādhimṛtyujarādibhiḥ ||38||

III.38: The yogi who remains even for half a twenty-four minutes (kṣaṇa) is freed from poisons, diseases that arise due to old age, and fear of death.

न रोगो मरणं तन्द्रा न निद्रा न क्षुधा तृषा ।
न च मूर्च्छा भवेत्तस्य यो मुद्रां वेत्ति खेचरीम् ॥३९॥

na rogo maraṇaṁ tandrā na nidrā na kṣudhā tṛṣā |
na ca mūrcchā bhavettasya yo mudrāṁ vetti khecarīm ||39||

III.39: There is no disease, death, laziness, sleep, hunger, thirst, or clouding of the intellect for the person who knows khecarī mudrā.

पीड्यते न स रोगेण लिप्यते न च कर्मणा ।
बाध्यते न स कालेन यो मुद्रां वेत्ति खेचरीम् ॥४०॥

pīḍyate na sa rogeṇa lipyate na ca karmaṇā |
bādhyate na sa kālena yo mudrāṁ vetti khecarīm ||40||

III.40: One who knows khecarī mudrā is not affected by disease, not tainted by karma, and not affected by time.

चित्तं चरति खे यस्माज्जिह्वा चरति खे गता ।
तेनैषा खेचरी नाम मुद्रा सिद्धैर्निरूपिता ॥४१ ॥

cittaṁ carati khe yasmājjihvā carati khe gatā |
tenaiṣā khecarī nāma mudrā siddhairnirūpitā ||41 ||

III.41: The adepts have named this mudrā "khecarī" because the mind moves in space [in the center of the eyebrows] and the tongue moves in the space [of the cavity behind the palate].

खेचर्या मुद्रितं येन विवरं लम्बिकोर्ध्वतः ।
न तस्य क्षरते बिन्दुः कामिन्या आश्लेषितस्य च ॥४२॥

khecaryā mudritaṁ yena vivaraṁ lambikordhvataḥ |
na tasya kṣarate binduḥ kāminyā āśleṣitasya ca ||42||

III.42: In one who has closed the cavity above the palate with the khecarī mudrā, seminal fluid is not wasted even when embraced by a passionate woman.

चलितोऽपि यदा बिन्दुः सम्प्राप्तो योनिमण्डलम् ।
व्रजत्यूर्ध्वं हृतः शक्त्या निबद्धो योनिमुद्रया ॥४३॥

calito'pi yadā binduḥ samprāpto yonimaṇḍalam |
vrajatyūrdhvaṁ hṛtaḥ śaktyā nibaddho yonimudrayā ||43||

III.43: Even if the seminal fluid flows down to the genitals (yoni), it is arrested by the yoni-mudrā and forced upwards.

ऊर्ध्वजिह्वः स्थिरो भूत्वा सोमपानं करोति यः ।
मासार्धेन न सन्देहो मृत्युं जयति योगवित् ॥४४॥

ūrdhvajihvaḥ sthiro bhūtvā somapānaṁ karoti yaḥ |
māsārdhena na sandeho mṛtyuṁ jayati yogavit ||44||

III.44: The knower of yoga, who, with steadiness, has the tongue turned upwards and drinks the nectar of the moon (soma), undoubtedly conquers death in a fortnight.

नित्यं सोमकलापूर्णं शरीरं यस्य योगिनः ।
तक्षकेणापि दष्टस्य विषं तस्य न सर्पति ॥४५॥

nityaṁ somakalāpūrṇaṁ śarīraṁ yasya yoginaḥ |
takṣakeṇāpi daṣṭasya viṣaṁ tasya na sarpati ||45||

III.45: In the body of a yogi, always imbued with nectar (soma), even when bitten by Takṣaka (one of the eight serpent kings), poison will not spread.

इन्धनानि यथा वह्निस्तैलवर्त्ति च दीपकः ।
तथा सोमकलापूर्णं देही देहं न मुञ्चति ॥४६॥

indhanāni yathā vahnistailavarttiṁ ca dīpakaḥ |
tathā somakalāpūrṇaṁ dehī dehaṁ na muñcati ||46||

III.46: As fire does not go out so long as there is fuel, as the light of a lamp does not die out so long as the wick has oil, so also the dweller does not desert the body that is filled by nectar of the moon (somakalā).

[Krishnamacharya] The idea is that the body will enter a hibernation state and all functions in the body will slow down.

गोमांसं भक्षयेन्नित्यं पिबेदमरवारुणीम् ।
कुलीनं तमहं मन्य इतरे कुलघातकाः ॥४७॥

gomāṁsaṁ bhakṣayennityaṁ pibedamaravāruṇīm |
kulīnaṁ tamahaṁ manya itare kulaghātakāḥ ||47||

III.47: I consider one who eats cow's meat (gomāṁsa) daily and drinks strong liquor (amaravāruṇī) to be well born. Others ruin [the reputation] of their family. (The words "gomāṁsa" and "amaravāruṇī" are explained in the next two verses).

गोशब्देनोदिता जिह्वा तत्प्रवेशो हि तालुनि ।
गोमांसभक्षणं तत्तु महापातकनाशनम् ॥४८॥

gośabdenoditā jihvā tatpraveśo hi tāluni |
gomāṁsabhakṣaṇaṁ tattu mahāpātakanāśanam ||48||

III.48: The word "go" refers to the tongue. Its entry into the cavity in the palate is eating the flesh of the cow (gomāṁsa-bhakṣaṇa). This destroys all the great sins.

जिह्वाप्रवेशसम्भूतवह्निनोत्पादितः खलु ।
चन्द्रात्स्रवति यः सारः सा स्यादमरवारुणी ॥४९॥

jihvāpraveśasambhūtavahninotpāditaḥ khalu |
candrātsravati yaḥ sāraḥ sā syādamaravāruṇī ||49||

III.49: The nectar which flows from the moon because of the heat produced by the entry of the tongue [into the cavity behind the palate] is called amaravāruṇī.

चुम्बन्ती यदि लम्बिकाग्रमनिशं जिह्वारसस्यन्दिनी
सक्षारा कटुकाम्लदुग्धसदृशी मध्वाज्यतुल्या तथा ।
व्याधीनां हरणं जरान्तकरणं शस्त्रागमोदीरणं
तस्य स्यादमरत्वमष्टगुणितं सिद्धाङ्गनाकर्षणम् ॥५०॥

cumbantī yadi lambikāgramaniśaṁ jihvārasasyandinī
sakṣārā kaṭukāmladugdhasadṛśī madhvājyatulyā tathā |

vyādhīnāṁ haraṇaṁ jarāntakaraṇaṁ śastrāgamodīraṇaṁ
tasya syādamaratvamaṣṭaguṇitaṁ siddhāṅganākarṣaṇam ||50||

III.50: If the tongue constantly touches the cavity in the palate, stimulating the flow of the nectar that tastes salty, pungent, and sour, like milk, honey, and ghee, all diseases are removed, aging is overcome, and weapons are warded off. Immortality and the eight special powers (siddhi-s) are attained and the divine damsels are attracted.

मूर्ध्नः षोडशपत्रपद्मगलितं प्राणादवाप्तं हठात्
ऊर्ध्वास्यो रसनां नियम्य विवरे शक्तिं परां चिन्तयन् ।
उत्कल्लोलकलाजलं च विमलं धारामयं यः पिबेत्
निर्व्याधिः स मृणालकोमलवपुर्योगी चिरं जीवति ॥५१॥

mūrdhnaḥ ṣoḍaśapatrapadmagalitaṁ prāṇādavāptaṁ haṭhāt
ūrdhvāsyo rasanāṁ niyamya vivare śaktiṁ parāṁ cintayan |
utkallolakalājalaṁ ca vimalaṁ dhārāmayaṁ yaḥ pibet
nirvyādhiḥ sa mṛṇālakomalavapuryogī ciraṁ jīvati ||51||

III.51: The yogi who, with upturned face and tongue closing the cavity of the palate, meditates on the supreme power (kuṇḍalinī) and drinks the clear nectar flowing in waves from the moon into the sixteen-petalled lotus [in the throat] through the control of prāṇa and the practice of haṭha-yoga, is freed from diseases and lives long with a body that is as soft and beautiful as the lotus stem.

यत्प्रालेयप्रहितसुषिरं मेरुमूर्धान्तरस्थं
तस्मिंस्तत्त्वं प्रवदति सुधीस्तन्मुखं निम्नगानाम् ।
चन्द्रात्सारः स्रवति वपुषस्तेन मृत्युर्नराणां
तद् बध्नीयात्सुकरणमतो नान्यथा कायसिद्धिः ॥५२॥

yatprāleyaprahitasuṣiraṁ merumūrdhāntarasthaṁ
tasmiṁstattvaṁ pravadati sudhīstanmukhaṁ nimnagānām |
candrātsāraḥ sravati vapuṣastena mṛtyurnarāṇāṁ
tadbadhnīyātsukaraṇamato nānyathā kāyasiddhiḥ ||52||

III.52: The nectar is within the cavity in the upper part of suṣumnā (meru). It is at the fountain-head of the nāḍī-s. One with a pure mind (sāttvika) will see that it is the place of truth (ātman, self). The nectar, the essence of the body, flows from the moon and death comes to man [when it is gone]. Therefore, one must practice the beneficial khecarī mudrā [to prevent its downward flow]. There is no other means to attain bodily mastery.

सुषिरं ज्ञानजनकं पञ्चस्रोतःसमन्वितम् ।
तिष्ठते खेचरी मुद्रा तस्मिञ्छून्ये निरञ्जने ॥५३॥

suṣiraṁ jñānajanakaṁ pañcasrotaḥsamanvitam |
tiṣṭhate khecarī mudrā tasmiñchūnye nirañjane ||53||

III.53: The cavity is the conjunction of the five streams and bestows Divine knowledge. In this space, untainted, the khecarī mudrā is firmly established.

[Krishnamacharya] The streams referred to are the many nāḍī-s (iḍā, piṅgalā, suṣumnā, gāndhārī etc.) which are, in the body, analogous to life-giving rivers such as Gangā, Yamunā, Sarasvatī, Narmadā etc. in a country.

एकं सृष्टिमयं बीजमेका मुद्रा च खेचरी ।
एको देवो निरालम्ब एकावस्था मनोन्मनी ॥५४॥

ekaṁ sṛṣṭimayaṁ bījamekā mudrā ca khecarī |
eko devo nirālamba ekāvasthā manonmanī ||54||

III.54: Most eminent among seeds (bija-s) is "OM," most eminent among mudrā-s is khecarī, most eminent among deities is one who is not dependent on anything (i.e. ātman or self), and the only worthy state of mind is manonmanī (samādhi).

[Krishnamacharya] Take the khecarī mudrā mentioned in this verse to be the one in Chapter IV, done along with prāṇāyāma, not the one here in Chapter III that involves cutting the frenulum of the tongue.

अथोड्डीयानबन्धः ।
बद्धो येन सुषुम्नायां प्राणस्तूड्डीयते यतः ।
तस्मादुड्डीयनाख्योऽयं योगिभिः समुदाहृतः ॥५५॥

athoḍḍīyānabandhaḥ |
baddho yena suṣumnāyāṁ prāṇastūḍḍīyate yataḥ |
tasmāduḍḍīyanākhyo'yaṁ yogibhiḥ samudāhṛtaḥ ||55||

Now uḍḍīyāna-bandha [is described].

III.55: Uḍḍīyāna-bandha is called so by the yogis, because when it is practiced, the prāṇa is controlled and flies through the suṣumnā.

[Krishnamacharya]

Practice uḍḍīyāna-bandha in tadāga-mudrā as a preparation.

Practice in chair pose (ardha-utkaṭāsana) holding upto 10 seconds. Use mantra to count the length of the breath. The practice should be done on an empty stomach. The feeling should be that the stomach joins the back bone.

With practice, in time, one should aim at suspension after exhalation for up to 32 seconds.

उड्डीनं कुरुते यस्मादविश्रान्तं महाखगः ।
उड्डीयानं तदेव स्यात्तत्र बन्धोऽभिधीयते ॥५६॥

uḍḍīnaṁ kurute yasmādaviśrāntaṁ mahākhagaḥ |
uḍḍīyānaṁ tadeva syāttatra bandho'bhidhīyate ||56||

III.56: This practice is called uḍḍīyāna-bandha, because through this the great bird (i.e. prāṇa) flies up without tiring [through the suṣumnā]. This bandha will now be explained.

[Krishnamacharya] All the three bandha-s are important for the practice of prāṇāyāma. When practicing uḍḍīyāna-bandha, one should have a feeling of inward pressure at the throat.

उदरे पश्चिमं तानं नाभेरूर्ध्वं च कारयेत् ।
उड्डीयानो ह्यसौ बन्धो मृत्युमातङ्गकेसरी ॥५७॥

udare paścimaṁ tānaṁ nābherūrdhvaṁ ca kārayet |
uḍḍīyāno hyasau bandho mṛtyumātaṅgakesarī ||57||

III.57: The drawing back of the abdomen above [and below] the navel is called uḍḍīyāna-bandha. This is the lion that kills the elephant of death.

[Krishnamacharya] Though the actual uḍḍīyāna-bandha is done after completing exhalation, mentally start the practice at the beginning of exhalation.

उड्डीयानं तु सहजं गुरुणा कथितं सदा ।
अभ्यसेत्सततं यस्तु वृद्धोऽपि तरुणायते ॥५८॥

uḍḍīyānaṁ tu sahajaṁ guruṇā kathitaṁ sadā |
abhyasetsatataṁ yastu vṛddho'pi taruṇāyate ||58||

III.58: When one continuously practices uḍḍīyāna-bandha as taught by the guru, doing it naturally, even if he is aged, he becomes young.

नाभेरूर्ध्वमधश्चापि तानं कुर्यात्प्रयत्नतः ।
षण्मासमभ्यसेन्मृत्युं जयत्येव न संशयः ॥५९॥

nābherūrdhvamadhaścāpi tānaṁ kuryātprayatnataḥ |
ṣaṇmāsamabhyasenmṛtyuṁ jayatyeva na saṁśayaḥ ||59||

III.59: With effort draw in [the abdomen] above and below the navel. By practicing for six months, death is conquered without a doubt.

[Krishnamacharya] "Death" here refers to an untimely death.

सर्वेषामेव बन्धानामुत्तमो ह्युड्डियानकः ।
उड्डियाने दृढे बन्धे मुक्तिः स्वाभाविकी भवेत् ॥६०॥

sarveṣāmeva bandhānāmuttamo hyuḍḍiyānakaḥ |
uḍḍiyāne dṛḍhe bandhe muktiḥ svābhāvikī bhavet ||60||

III.60: Of all the bandha-s, uḍḍīyāna is said to be the best. When this has been mastered, liberation follows naturally.

[Krishnamacharya] Liberation can also be taken to mean freedom from disease, and a state of good health, which becomes natural.

When uḍḍīyāna-bandha has been mastered, the prāṇa flows through the suṣumnā and reaches the crown of the head (brahmarandhra). Samādhi is attained by this practice, which can in turn lead to liberation (mokṣa).

अथ मूलबन्धः ।
पार्ष्णिभागेन संपीड्य योनिमाकुञ्चयेद्गुदम् ।
अपानमूर्ध्वमाकृष्य मूलबन्धोऽभिधीयते ॥६१॥

atha mūlabandhaḥ |
pārṣṇibhāgena saṁpīḍya yonimākuñcayedgudam |
apānamūrdhvamākṛṣya mūlabandho'bhidhīyate ||61||

Now mūla-bandha [is described].

III.61: Pressing the perineum with the heel, contract the perineum and draw the apāna upwards. This is known as mūla-bandha.

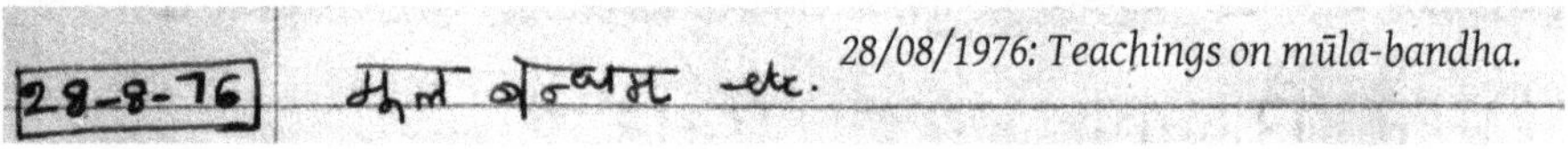

28/08/1976: Teachings on mūla-bandha.

[Krishnamacharya] Gheraṇḍa Saṁhitā III.14-15 also describes mūla-bandha. However, the description given in verse III.14 as mūla-bandha is in fact mūla-bandha-mudrā and not just mūla-bandha. Mūla-bandhāsana, mūla-bandha-mudrā, and mūla-bandha are not the same. Mūla-bandha-mudrā is useful for siddhi (success) of mūla-bandha.

Practice mūla-bandha first in headstand before trying it out in seated postures.

अधोगतिमपानं वा ऊर्ध्वगं कुरुते बलात् ।
आकुञ्चनेन तं प्राहुर्मूलबन्धं हि योगिनः ॥६२॥

adhogatimapānaṁ vā ūrdhvagaṁ kurute balāt |
ākuñcanena taṁ prāhurmūlabandhaṁ hi yoginaḥ ||62||

III.62: By forceful contraction [of the mūlādhāra] the downward moving apāna is forced to go upwards [through suṣumnā]. Yogins call this mūla-bandha.

[Krishnamacharya] All the nāḍī-s start from mūlādhāra (root of the pelvis). The mūlādhāra mentioned here may also be referred to as kanda.

गुदं पार्ष्ण्या तु सम्पीड्य वायुमाकुञ्चयेद्बलात् ।
वारं वारं यथा चोर्ध्वं समायाति समीरणः ॥६३॥

gudaṁ pārṣṇyā tu sampīḍya vāyumākuñcayedbalāt |
vāraṁ vāraṁ yathā cordhvaṁ samāyāti samīraṇaḥ ||63||

III.63: Pressing the perineum with the heel, contract the breath (apāna) forcibly and repeatedly till the breath (apāna) moves upwards. [This is mūla-bandha.]

प्राणापानौ नादबिन्दू मूलबन्धेन चैकताम् ।
गत्वा योगस्य संसिद्धिं यच्छतो नात्र संशयः ॥६४॥

prāṇāpānau nādabindū mūlabandhena caikatām |
gatvā yogasya saṁsiddhiṁ yacchato nātra saṁśayaḥ ||64||

III.64: Through the practice of mūla-bandha, prāṇa and apāna unite with nāda and bindu and bestow perfection in yoga. There is no doubt about this.

[Krishnamacharya] Nāda here refers to nādānusandhāna or hearing the inner sound. Bindu refers to vitality.

There are two Upaniṣats known as Nādabindu Upaniṣat and Amṛtabindu Upaniṣat.

All the five prāṇa-s join and become one; that is, they enter suṣumnā.

अपानप्राणयोरैक्यं क्षयो मूत्रपुरीषयोः ।
युवा भवति वृद्धोऽपि सततं मूलबन्धनात् ॥६५॥

apānaprāṇayoraikyaṁ kṣayo mūtrapurīṣayoḥ |
yuvā bhavati vṛddho'pi satataṁ mūlabandhanāt ||65||

III.65: Through the continuous practice of mūla-bandha, prāṇa and apāna unite. Urine and excrement decrease and even an aged person becomes young.

[Krishnamacharya] The practice protects against old age diseases of bowel movement and urination.

अपान ऊर्ध्वगे जाते प्रयाते वह्निमण्डलम् ।
तदानलशिखा दीर्घा जायते वायुनाहता ॥६६॥

apāna ūrdhvage jāte prayāte vahnimaṇḍalam |
tadānalaśikhā dīrghā jāyate vāyunāhatā ||66||

III.66: When apāna rises upwards and reaches the sphere of fire, the flame of the fire lengthens, fanned by apāna.

[Krishnamacharya] According to the Yoga Yājñavalkya, the sphere of the fire is said to be triangular in humans and its place is in the center of the body, below the navel. In quadrupeds it is rectangular, and in birds it is circular.

ततो यातो वह्न्यपानौ प्राणमुष्णस्वरूपकम् ।
तेनात्यन्तप्रदीप्तस्तु ज्वलनो देहजस्तथा ॥६७॥

tato yāto vahnyapānau prāṇamuṣṇasvarūpakam |
tenātyantapradīptastu jvalano dehajastathā ||67||

III.67: Then the apāna and the fire join prāṇa which is hot by nature. This greatly intensifies the heat in the body.

[Krishnamacharya] Refer Yoga Yājñavalkya.

तेन कुण्डलिनी सुप्ता सन्तप्ता सम्प्रबुध्यते ।
दण्डाहता भुजङ्गीव निश्वस्य ऋजुतां व्रजेत् ॥६८॥

tena kuṇḍalinī suptā santaptā samprabudhyate |
daṇḍāhatā bhujaṅgīva niśvasya ṛjutāṁ vrajet ||68||

III.68: Thus scorched, the sleeping kuṇḍalinī awakens. Like a snake struck by a stick, it hisses and straightens itself.

बिलं प्रविष्टेव ततो ब्रह्मनाड्यन्तरं व्रजेत् ।
तस्मान्नित्यं मूलबन्धः कर्तव्यो योगिभिः सदा ॥६९॥

bilaṁ praviṣṭeva tato brahmanāḍyantaraṁ vrajet |
tasmānnityaṁ mūlabandhaḥ kartavyo yogibhiḥ sadā ||69||

III.69: Then, like a [snake] entering its burrow, it (kuṇḍalinī) enters the suṣumnā (brahmanāḍī). Therefore, yogis should practice mūla-bandha every day.

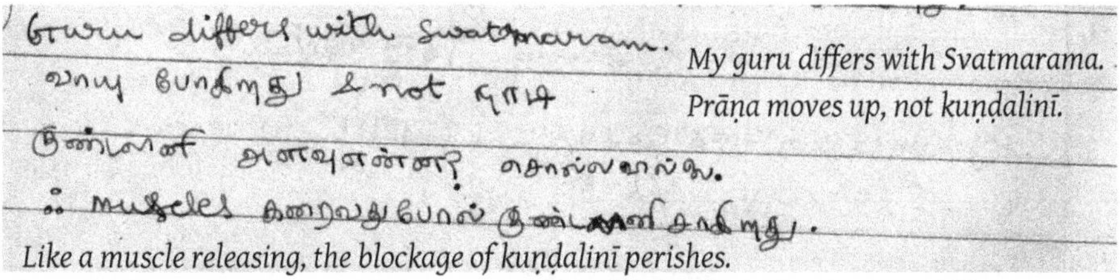
Guru differs with Swatmaram.
My guru differs with Svatmarama.
Prāṇa moves up, not kuṇḍalinī.
Like a muscle releasing, the blockage of kuṇḍalinī perishes.

[Krishnamacharya] This means that the mind becomes completely focused.

अथ जालन्धरबन्धः ।
कण्ठमाकुञ्च्य हृदये स्थापयेच्चिबुकं दृढम् ।
बन्धो जालन्धराख्योऽयं जरामृत्युविनाशकः ॥७०॥

atha jālandharabandhaḥ |
kaṇṭhamākuñcya hṛdaye sthāpayeccibukaṁ dṛḍham |
bandho jālandharākhyo'yaṁ jarāmṛtyuvināśakaḥ ||70||

Now jālandhara-bandha [is described].

III.70: Contracting the throat, hold the chin firmly against the chest. This is called jālandhara-bandha which destroys aging and death.

[Krishnamacharya] The word jālandhara is from "jala" meaning "liquid" and "dhara" meaning "to hold." The implication of the word "liquid" is that it has a tendency to spread. The reference is not to liquid, but to all sensations and sensory inputs, which spread from the senses in the head, and from there, into the body. Since the head holds all the sensations, the head itself is called jālandhara. The word bandha, as noted earlier, means "to bind." Thus, this bandha helps to bind the essence of all the sensations.

Postures like dvipādapīṭham and uttāna-mayūrāsana with proper breathing are helpful for jālandhara-bandha.

बध्नाति हि सिराजालमधोगामि नभोजलम् ।
ततो जालन्धरो बन्धः कण्ठदुःखौघनाशनः ॥७१॥

badhnāti hi sirājālamadhogāmi nabhojalam |
tato jālandharo bandhaḥ kaṇṭhaduḥkhaughanāśanaḥ ||71||

III.71: Because it constricts the network of nāḍī-s and [arrests] the downward flow of ambrosial nectar [from the cavity in the palate], it is called jālandhara. It wards off all maladies of the throat.

जालन्धरे कृते बन्धे कण्ठसङ्कोचलक्षणे ।
न पीयूषं पतत्यग्नौ न च वायुः प्रकुप्यति ॥७२॥

jālandhare kṛte bandhe kaṇṭhasaṅkocalakṣaṇe |
na pīyūṣaṁ patatyagnau na ca vāyuḥ prakupyati ||72||

III.72: When jālandhara-bandha is practiced, by contracting the throat, the nectar does not fall into the [gastric] fire and prāṇa is not misdirected.

कण्ठसङ्कोचनेनैव द्वे नाड्यौ स्तम्भयेद्दृढम् ।
मध्यचक्रमिदं ज्ञेयं षोडशाधारबन्धनम् ॥७३॥

kaṇṭhasaṅkocanenaiva dve nāḍyau stambhayeddṛḍham |
madhyacakramidaṁ jñeyaṁ ṣoḍaśādhārabandhanam ||73||

III.73: By [firmly] contracting the throat, the two nāḍī-s [iḍā and piṅgalā] are made inert. Here [in the throat] is situated the middle cakra (viśuddhi). This binds the sixteen vital centers (ādhāra-s).

मूलस्थानं समाकुञ्च्य उड्डियानं तु कारयेत् ।
इडां च पिङ्गलां बद्ध्वा वाहयेत्पश्चिमे पथि ॥७४॥

mūlasthānaṁ samākuñcya uḍḍiyānaṁ tu kārayet |
iḍāṁ ca piṅgalāṁ baddhvā vāhayetpaścime pathi ||74 ||

III.74: Contracting the foundation (i.e. the pelvic floor with mūla-bandha), practice the uḍḍīyāna-bandha. Constrain the iḍā and piṅgalā and enable [prāṇa] to flow through the suṣumnā.

अनेनैव विधानेन प्रयाति पवनो लयम् ।
ततो न जायते मृत्युर्जरारोगादिकं तथा ॥७५॥

anenaiva vidhānena prayāti pavano layam |
tato na jāyate mṛtyurjarārogādikaṁ tathā ||75||

III.75: Through these means, the prāṇa becomes steady [in suṣumnā]. Then there is no fear of death, aging and disease, etc.

[Krishnamacharya] The practice of prāṇāyāma with the three bandha-s leads to kevala-kumbhaka.

बन्धत्रयमिदं श्रेष्ठं महासिद्धैश्च सेवितम् ।
सर्वेषां हठतन्त्राणां साधनं योगिनो विदुः ॥७६॥

bandhatrayamidaṁ śreṣṭhaṁ mahāsiddhaiśca sevitam |
sarveṣāṁ haṭhatantrāṇāṁ sādhanaṁ yogino viduḥ ||76||

III.76: These three excellent bandha-s have been practiced by the great adepts (siddha-s). Yogi-s consider them fundamental to various haṭha-yoga practices.

यत्किञ्चित्स्रवते चन्द्रादमृतं दिव्यरूपिणः ।
तत्सर्वं ग्रसते सूर्यस्तेन पिण्डो जरायुतः ॥७७॥

yatkiñcitsravate candrādamṛtaṁ divyarūpiṇaḥ |
tatsarvaṁ grasate sūryastena piṇḍo jarāyutaḥ ||77||

III.77: All the nectar that flows from the moon (candra) which is of divine form, is consumed by gastric fire (surya). Hence the body grows old.

[Krishnamacharya] Viparītakaraṇī, sarvaṅgāsana, and śīrṣāsana fall under the same category and should be learned in that order. However, after becoming adept at practicing them, headstand is done before shoulderstand in a sequence. Headstand helps in mūla-bandha and uḍḍīyāna-bandha. In shoulderstand, all the three bandha-s can be practiced. Classically, these inversions are followed by mahāmudrā. The three bandha-s are usually done along with jihvā-bandha in mahāmudrā.

अथ विपरीतकरणी मुद्रा ।
तत्रास्ति करणं दिव्यं सूर्यस्य मुखवञ्चनम् ।
गुरूपदेशतो ज्ञेयं न तु शास्त्रार्थकोटिभिः ॥७८॥

atha viparītakaraṇī mudrā |
tatrāsti karaṇaṁ divyaṁ sūryasya mukhavañcanam |
gurūpadeśato jñeyaṁ na tu śāstrārthakoṭibhiḥ ||78||

Now viparītakaraṇī mudrā [is described].

III.78: There is an excellent process by which the mouth of the sun is cheated. This should be learnt from a guru and not through theoretical study of the texts.

ऊर्ध्वनाभेरधस्तालोरूर्ध्वं भानुरधः शशी ।
करणी विपरीताख्या गुरुवाक्येन लभ्यते ॥७९॥

ūrdhvanābheradhastālorūrdhvaṁ bhānuradhaḥ śaśī |
karaṇī viparītākhyā guruvākyena labhyate ||79||

III.79: When [the practitioner assumes a position] where the navel is above and the palate is below, where the sun is above and the moon is below, it is called viparītakaraṇī. It is to be learnt through the instructions of a guru.

नित्यमभ्यासयुक्तस्य जठराग्निविवर्धिनी ।
आहारो बहुलस्तस्य सम्पाद्यः साधकस्य च ॥८०॥

nityamabhyāsayuktasya jaṭharāgnivivardhinī |
āhāro bahulastasya sampādyaḥ sādhakasya ca ||80||

III.80: In one who practices this [viparītakaraṇī] daily, the gastric fire is increased and the practitioner should be provided with plenty of food.

अल्पाहारो यदि भवेदग्निर्दहति तत्क्षणात् ।
अधःशिराश्चोर्ध्वपादः क्षणं स्यात्प्रथमे दिने ॥८१॥

alpāhāro yadi bhavedagnirdahati tatkṣaṇāt |
adhaḥśirāścordhvapādaḥ kṣaṇaṁ syātprathame dine ||81||

III.81: If he takes a small quantity of food, the fire quickly consumes [the body]. The head is placed on the ground and the legs are raised above. This position should be held only for a moment on the first day.

क्षणाच्च किञ्चिदधिकमभ्यसेच्च दिने दिने ।
वलितं पलितं चैव षण्मासोर्ध्वं न दृश्यते ।
याममात्रं तु यो नित्यमभ्यसेत् स तु कालजित् ॥८२॥

kṣaṇācca kiñcidadhikamabhyasecca dine dine |
valitaṁ palitaṁ caiva ṣaṇmāsordhvaṁ na dṛśyate |
yāmamātraṁ tu yo nityamabhyaset sa tu kālajit ||82||

III.82: Practice this by gradually increasing the duration each day. Wrinkles and grey hair disappear after six months. If this is practiced daily only for three hours (yamā-mātra) fear of death is conquered.

अथ वज्रोली ।
स्वेच्छया वर्तमानोऽपि योगोक्तैर्नियमैर्विना ।
वज्रोलीं यो विजानाति स योगी सिद्धिभाजनम् ॥८३॥

atha vajrolī |
svecchayā vartamāno'pi yogoktairniyamairvinā |
vajrolīṁ yo vijānāti sa yogī siddhibhājanam ||83||

Now vajrolī [is described].

III.83: Even a person leading an unrestricted life, without the discipline prescribed by yoga, if he knows vajrolī well (i.e. is adept at it), becomes the repository of the special powers (siddhi-s).

[Krishnamacharya] described the practice in my studies with him (see notes under IV.86 below), but he also noted that the practice is neither useful for oneself nor for others.

"Vajra" means "diamond." The idea is that the body becomes like a diamond through the practice of celibacy. The way this practice is structured and described, it is mainly aimed at cultivating and testing a physical skill.

तत्र वस्तुद्वयं वक्ष्ये दुर्लभं यस्य कस्यचित् ।
क्षीरं चैकं द्वितीयं तु नारी च वशवर्तिनी ॥८४॥

tatra vastudvayaṁ vakṣye durlabhaṁ yasya kasyacit |
kṣīraṁ caikaṁ dvitīyaṁ tu nārī ca vaśavartinī ||84||

III.84: I must mention that two things are difficult for the practitioner [of vajrolī] to obtain. One is milk [at the proper time] and the other, a woman who will comply with one's wishes.

मेहनेन शनैः सम्यगूर्ध्वाकुञ्चनमभ्यसेत् ।
पुरुषोऽप्यथवा नारी वज्रोलीसिद्धिमाप्नुयात् ॥८५॥

mehanena śanaiḥ samyagūrdhvākuñcanamabhyaset |
puruṣo'pyathavā nārī vajrolīsiddhimāpnuyāt ||85 ||

III.85: At the time of [emission of seminal fluid during] sexual intercourse, practice to draw it up slowly. This is the way by which a man or a woman will attain success in vajrolī.

यत्नतः शस्तनालेन फूत्कारं वज्रकन्दरे ।
शनैः शनैः प्रकुर्वीत वायुसञ्चारकारणात् ॥८६॥

yatnataḥ śastanālena phūtkāraṁ vajrakandare |
śanaiḥ śanaiḥ prakurvīta vāyusañcārakāraṇāt ||86||

III.86: Insert the prescribed tube into the opening of the penis and blow through it to allow the passage of air.

[Krishnamacharya] Preparing for vajrolī.

Practice tadāga-mudrā seated in paścimatānāsana (ref: Gheraṇḍa Saṁhitā III.61).

Practice tadāga-mudrā in upaviṣṭakoṇāsana.

Practice mūla-bandha.

Practice uḍḍīyāna-bandha and mūla-bandha in upaviṣṭakoṇāsana.

Sit with legs spread and back straight with jālandhara-bandha to cleanse the tube.

नारीभगे पतद्बिन्दुमभ्यासेनोर्ध्वमाहरेत् ।
चलितं च निजं बिन्दुमूर्ध्वमाकृष्य रक्षयेत् ॥८७॥

nārībhage patadbindumabhyāsenordhvamāharet |
calitaṁ ca nijaṁ bindumūrdhvamākṛṣya rakṣayet ||87||

III.87: The semen that is about to drop into the genitals of a woman should be drawn up by practice [of vajrolī]. If already fallen, he should draw up the semen and preserve it.

एवं संरक्षयेद्बिन्दुं मृत्युं जयति योगवित् ।
मरणं बिन्दुपातेन जीवनं बिन्दुधारणात् ॥८८॥

evaṁ saṁrakṣayedbinduṁ mṛtyuṁ jayati yogavit |
maraṇaṁ bindupātena jīvanaṁ bindudhāraṇāt ||88||

III.88: The knower of yoga, by preserving his semen, conquers death. When the semen is expended, death ensues [in due course]. There is prolonged life for one who preserves it.

सुगन्धो योगिनो देहे जायते बिन्दुधारणात् ।
यावद्बिन्दुः स्थिरो देहे तावत्कालभयं कुतः ॥८९॥

sugandho yogino dehe jāyate bindudhāraṇāt |
yāvadbinduḥ sthiro dehe tāvatkālabhayaṁ kutaḥ ||89||

III.89: Preserving the semen [by the vajrolī] gives rise to a pleasant smell in the body of the yogi. As long as the semen is well retained in the body, where is the fear of death?

चित्तायत्तं नृणां शुक्रं शुक्रायत्तं च जीवितम् ।
तस्माच्छुक्रं मनश्चैव रक्षणीयं प्रयत्नतः ॥९०॥

cittāyattaṁ nṛṇāṁ śukraṁ śukrāyattaṁ ca jīvitam |
tasmācchukraṁ manaścaiva rakṣaṇīyaṁ prayatnataḥ ||90||

III.90: The retention of semen is controlled by the mind and [long] life depends on the semen. Therefore, both mind and semen should be carefully preserved.

ऋतुमत्या रजोऽप्येवं निजं बिन्दुं च रक्षयेत् ।
मेढ्रेणाकर्षयेदूर्ध्वं सम्यगभ्यासयोगवित् ॥९१॥

ṛtumatyā rajo'pyevaṁ nijaṁ binduṁ ca rakṣayet |
meḍhreṇākarṣayedūrdhvaṁ samyagabhyāsayogavit ||91||

III.91: A person who is an expert in this practice should preserve his seminal fluid and that of the woman with whom he has intercourse, by drawing them up well through the penis.

अथ सहजोलिः ।
सहजोलिश्चामरोलिर्वज्रोल्या भेद एकतः ।
जलेषु भस्म निक्षिप्य दग्धगोमयसम्भवम् ॥९२॥
वज्रोलीमैथुनादूर्ध्वं स्त्रीपुंसोः स्वाङ्गलेपनम् ।
आसीनयोः सुखेनैव मुक्तव्यापारयोः क्षणात् ॥९३॥

atha sahajoliḥ |
sahajoliścāmarolirvajrolyā bheda ekataḥ |
jaleṣu bhasma nikṣipya dagdhagomayasambhavam ||92||

vajrolīmaithunādūrdhvaṁ strīpuṁsoḥ svāṅgalepanam |
āsīnayoḥ sukhenaiva muktavyāpārayoḥ kṣaṇāt ||93||

Now sahajolī [is described].

III.92-93: Sahajolī and amarolī are varieties of vajrolī since they are one [in respect to results attained]. Mix the ash of cow-dung with water. Soon after intercourse with vajrolī, the man and woman, sitting with a relaxed frame of mind, should smear [this mixture] on the parts of the body.

सहजोलिरियं प्रोक्ता श्रद्धेया योगिभिः सदा ।
अयं शुभकरो योगो भोगयुक्तोऽपि मुक्तिदः ॥९४॥

sahajoliriyaṁ proktā śraddheyā yogibhiḥ sadā |
ayaṁ śubhakaro yogo bhogayukto'pi muktidaḥ ||94||

III.94: This is sahajolī which should be regarded with confidence by yogis. It is a beneficial practice and bestows liberation though connected with sensual experience.

अयं योगः पुण्यवतां धीराणां तत्त्वदर्शिनाम् ।
निर्मत्सराणां वै सिध्येत न तु मत्सरशालिनाम् ॥९५॥

ayaṁ yogaḥ puṇyavatāṁ dhīrāṇāṁ tattvadarśinām |
nirmatsarāṇāṁ vai sidhyeta na tu matsaraśālinām ||95||

III.95: This yoga practice succeeds only for those who are virtuous, who are brave, who perceive the truth, and who are free from envy. Envious persons will not succeed.

अथामरोली ।
पित्तोल्बणत्वात् प्रथमाम्बुधारां विहाय निःसारतयान्त्यधाराम् ।
निषेव्यते शीतलमध्यधारा कापालिके खण्डमतेऽमरोली ॥९६॥

athāmarolī |
pittolbaṇatvāt prathamāmbudhārāṁ vihāya niḥsāratayāntyadhārām |
niṣevyate śītalamadhyadhārā kāpālike khaṇḍamate'marolī ||96||

Now amarolī [is described]:

III.96: Discarding the first part of the flow [of amarī] (i.e. urine) as it increases bile, and the last flow as being without essence, when the cool middle part of the stream [of urine] is absorbed, this is amarolī according to the kāpālika sect.

अमरीं यः पिबेन्नित्यं नस्यं कुर्वन्दिने दिने ।
वज्रोलीमभ्यसेत्सम्यक् सामरोलीति कथ्यते ॥९७॥

amarīṁ yaḥ pibennityaṁ nasyaṁ kurvandine dine |
vajrolīmabhyasetsamyak sāmarolīti kathyate ||97||

III.97: One who drinks amarī (urine) daily and inhales it every day, should practice vajrolī well. This is called amarolī.

अभ्यासान्निःसृतां चान्द्रीं विभूत्या सह मिश्रयेत् ।
धारयेदुत्तमाङ्गेषु दिव्यदृष्टिः प्रजायते ॥९८॥

abhyāsānniḥsṛtāṁ cāndrīṁ vibhūtyā saha miśrayet |
dhārayeduttamāṅgeṣu divyadṛṣṭiḥ prajāyate ||98||

III.98: One should mix with ash the nectar flowing from the moon due to the practice [of amarolī] and smear it on the principal limbs. This leads to divine sight.

पुंसो बिन्दुं समाकुञ्च्य सम्यगभ्यासपाटवात् ।
यदि नारी रजो रक्षेद्वज्रोल्या सापि योगिनी ॥९९ ॥

puṁso binduṁ samākuñcya samyagabhyāsapāṭavāt |
yadi nārī rajo rakṣedvajrolyā sāpi yoginī ||99 ||

III.99: If a woman, through the expertise in the practice of vajrolī, draws up the semen of the man and preserves it with her own, she too becomes a yoginī.

तस्याः किञ्चिद्रजो नाशं न गच्छति न संशयः ।
तस्याः शरीरे नादश्च बिन्दुतामेव गच्छति ॥१००॥

tasyāḥ kiñcidrajo nāśaṁ na gacchati na saṁśayaḥ |
tasyāḥ śarīre nādaśca bindutāmeva gacchati ||100||

III.100: There is no doubt that even the least part of her fluid is not lost. In her body, the nāda becomes bindu itself.

स बिन्दुस्तद्रजश्चैव एकीभूय स्वदेहगौ ।
वज्रोल्यभ्यासयोगेन सर्वसिद्धिं प्रयच्छतः ॥१०१॥

sa bindustadrajaścaiva ekībhūya svadehagau |
vajrolyabhyāsayogena sarvasiddhiṁ prayacchataḥ ||101||

III.101: That semen and fluid, uniting and remaining in the body through the practice of vajrolī, confer all special powers (siddhi-s).

रक्षेदाकुञ्चनादूर्ध्वं या रजः सा हि योगिनी ।
अतीतानागतं वेत्ति खेचरी च भवेद्ध्रुवम् ॥१०२॥

rakṣedākuñcanādūrdhvaṁ yā rajaḥ sā hi yoginī |
atītānāgataṁ vetti khecarī ca bhaveddhruvam ||102||

III.102: She who preserves her fluid by drawing it upwards is a yoginī. She knows the past and future and certainly attains khecarī.

देहसिद्धिं च लभते वज्रोल्यभ्यासयोगतः ।
अयं पुण्यकरो योगो भोगे भुक्तेऽपि मुक्तिदः ॥१०३॥

dehasiddhiṁ ca labhate vajrolyabhyāsayogataḥ |
ayaṁ puṇyakaro yogo bhoge bhukte'pi muktidaḥ ||103||

III.103: The practice of vajrolī also results in bodily perfection. This yoga confers merit (puṇya) and although there is sensual experience, it leads to liberation.

अथ शक्तिचालनम् ।
कुटिलाङ्गी कुण्डलिनी भुजङ्गी शक्तिरीश्वरी ।
कुण्दल्यरुन्धती चैते शब्दाः पर्यायवाचकाः ॥१०४॥

atha śakticālanam |
kuṭilāṅgī kuṇḍalinī bhujaṅgī śaktirīśvarī |
kuṇḍalyarundhatī caite śabdāḥ paryāyavācakāḥ ||104||

Now śakti-cālana [is described].

III.104: Kutilāṅgi, Kuṇḍalinī, Bhujaṅgi, Śakti, Īśvarī, Kuṇḍalī, and Arundhatī are all synonymous words.

[Krishnamacharya] The practice of śakti-cālana involves forceful methods; it is risky and non-essential. In haṭha-yoga practice, kuṇḍalinī is a nāḍī to be controlled. There is only one śakti or energy in us and that is prāṇa. How can there be another śakti called kuṇḍalinī? We use prāṇa to move kuṇḍalinī. In the śākta tradition, kuṇḍalinī is considered the deity of prāṇa. The approach there is different.

उद्घाटयेत्कपाटं तु यथा कुञ्चिकया हठात् ।
कुण्डलिन्या तथा योगी मोक्षद्वारं विभेदयेत् ॥१०५॥

udghāṭayetkapāṭaṁ tu yathā kuñcikayā haṭhāt |
kuṇḍalinyā tathā yogī mokṣadvāraṁ vibhedayet ||105||

III.105: Just as one uses a key to open a door, so too the yogi should through the practice of haṭha-yoga, open the door of liberation with the power of kuṇḍalinī.

[Krishnamacharya] This is a simile. Just as a key is turned to open a door, prāṇa is used to move the kuṇḍalinī, so that prāṇa can enter suṣumnā. The door is kuṇḍalinī and the key is mastering the prāṇa through haṭha-yoga.

येन मार्गेण गन्तव्यं ब्रह्मस्थानं निरामयम् ।
मुखेनाच्छाद्य तद्वारं प्रसुप्ता परमेश्वरी ॥१०६॥

yena mārgeṇa gantavyaṁ brahmasthānaṁ nirāmayam |
mukhenācchādya taddvāraṁ prasuptā parameśvarī ||106||

III.106: The great goddess [kuṇḍalinī] sleeps, closing with her mouth the entrance to the abode of Brahman, free of all pain.

कन्दोर्ध्वे कुण्डली शक्तिः सुप्ता मोक्षाय योगिनाम् ।
बन्धनाय च मूढानां यस्तां वेत्ति स योगवित् ॥१०७॥

kandordhve kuṇḍalī śaktiḥ suptā mokṣāya yogināṃ |
bandhanāya ca mūḍhānāṁ yastāṁ vetti sa yogavit ||107||

III.107: The power (śakti) of kuṇḍalinī, who sleeps above the kanda, bestows liberation on yogis and bondage on the ignorant. One who knows her is the knower of yoga.

[Krishnamacharya] Refer the Yoga Yājñavalkya, Chapter IV, for a detailed description of the kanda and other related information.

कुण्डली कुटिलाकारा सर्पवत्परिकीर्तिता ।
सा शक्तिश्चालिता येन स मुक्तो नात्र संशयः ॥१०८॥

kuṇḍalī kuṭilākārā sarpavatparikīrtitā |
sā śaktiścālitā yena sa mukto nātra saṁśayaḥ ||108||

III.108: Kuṇḍalinī is described, as being coiled like a snake. One who is able to move that power (śakti) [from the mūlādhāra upwards] is liberated without doubt.

[Krishnamacharya] This verse describes the shape of the kuṇḍalinī. The kuṇḍalinī blocks the flow of prāṇa and prevents the prāṇa from entering suṣumnā.

गङ्गायमुनयोर्मध्ये बालरण्डां तपस्विनीम् ।
बलात्कारेण गृह्णीयात्तद्विष्णोः परमं पदम् ॥१०९॥

gaṅgāyamunayormadhye bālaraṇḍāṁ tapasvinīm |
balātkāreṇa gṛhṇīyāttadviṣṇoḥ paramaṁ padam ||109||

III.109: Between the Gangā and the Yamunā, a young widow (kuṇḍalinī) practices austerities. She should be seized forcefully. This [leads to] the supreme seat of Lord Viṣṇu.

इडा भगवती गङ्गा पिङ्गला यमुना नदी ।
इडापिङ्गलयोर्मध्ये बालरण्डा च कुण्डली ॥ ११० ॥

iḍā bhagavatī gaṅgā piṅgalā yamunā nadī |
iḍāpiṅgalayormadhye bālaraṇḍā ca kuṇḍalī ||110||

III.110: Iḍā is the goddess Gangā and piṅgalā is the river Yamunā. Between Iḍā and Piṅgalā is the young widow Kuṇḍalinī.

पुच्छे प्रगृह्य भुजगीं सुप्तामुद्बोधयेच्च ताम् ।
निद्रां विहाय सा शक्तिरूर्ध्वमुत्तिष्ठते हठात् ॥ १११ ॥

pucche pragṛhya bhujagīṁ suptāmudbodhayecca tām |
nidrāṁ vihāya sā śaktirūrdhvamuttiṣṭhate haṭhāt ||111||

III.111: By seizing the tail of the sleeping serpent (kuṇḍalinī), she should be awakened. Then, that power (śakti), throwing off her sleep, rises upwards with great force.

[Krishnamacharya] This verse starts the description of the practice of śakti-cālana. The word haṭha here refers not to force, but to the practice of prāṇāyāma.

अवस्थिता चैव फणावती सा प्रातश्च सायं प्रहरार्धमात्रम् ।
प्रपूर्य सूर्यात्परिधानयुक्त्या प्रगृह्य नित्यं परिचालनीया ॥ ११२ ॥

avasthitā caiva phaṇāvatī sā prātaśca sāyaṁ praharārdhamātram |
prapūrya sūryātparidhānayuktyā pragṛhya nityaṁ paricālanīyā ||112||

III.112: After inhaling through the right nostril, the serpent below should be grasped through the process of paridhāna, and moved daily, morning and evening, for an hour and a half.

[Krishnamacharya] Through specific practices of nauli, known as paridhāna, one can experience the kanda, located four angula-s (finger widths) below the navel.

ऊर्ध्वं वितस्तिमात्रं तु विस्तारं चतुरङ्गुलम् ।
मृदुलं धवलं प्रोक्तं वेष्टिताम्बरलक्षणम् ॥११३॥

ūrdhvaṁ vitastimātraṁ tu vistāraṁ caturaṅgulam |
mṛdulaṁ dhavalaṁ proktaṁ veṣṭitāmbaralakṣaṇam ||113||

III.113: The kanda is located twelve angula-s (finger widths) above the perineum and is four angula-s in breadth. It is said to be soft and white, like a rolled cloth.

सति वज्रासने पादौ कराभ्यां धारयेद्दृढम् ।
गुल्फदेशसमीपे च कन्दं तत्र प्रपीडयेत् ॥११४॥

sati vajrāsane pādau karābhyāṁ dhārayeddṛḍham |
gulphadeśasamīpe ca kandaṁ tatra prapīḍayet ||114||

III.114: Seated firmly in vajrāsana, hold near the ankles firmly with the hands, thereby putting pressure on the kanda.

[Krishnamacharya] The posture is sitting back on the heels.

वज्रासने स्थितो योगी चालयित्वा च कुण्डलीम् ।
कुर्यादनन्तरं भस्त्रां कुण्डलीमाशु बोधयेत् ॥११५॥

vajrāsane sthito yogī cālayitvā ca kuṇḍalīm |
kuryādanantaraṁ bhastrāṁ kuṇḍalīmāśu bodhayet ||115||

III.115: Seated in vajrāsana, the yogi having moved the kuṇḍalinī, should then practice bhastrikā (fast breathing). This will quickly awaken the kuṇḍalinī.

[Krishnamacharya] Engage mūla-bandha mildly and practice rapid inhale and exhale. The body may tend to lean forward a little, so hold the ankles to keep upright.

भानोराकुञ्चनं कुर्यात्कुण्डलीं चालयेत्ततः ।
मृत्युवक्त्रगतस्यापि तस्य मृत्युभयं कुतः ॥११६॥

bhānorākuñcanaṁ kuryātkuṇḍalīṁ cālayettataḥ |
mṛtyuvaktragatasyāpi tasya mṛtyubhayaṁ kutaḥ ||116||

III.116: Then contract the sun (which is near the navel) and move the kuṇḍalinī towards it. [Doing thus,] even when death approaches, he (the yogi) will have no fear of death.

[Krishnamacharya] The order of the practice should be as follows:

Do mūla-bandha, uḍḍīyāna-bandha, and nauli. With practice, the nauli will taper toward the lower part of the abdomen.

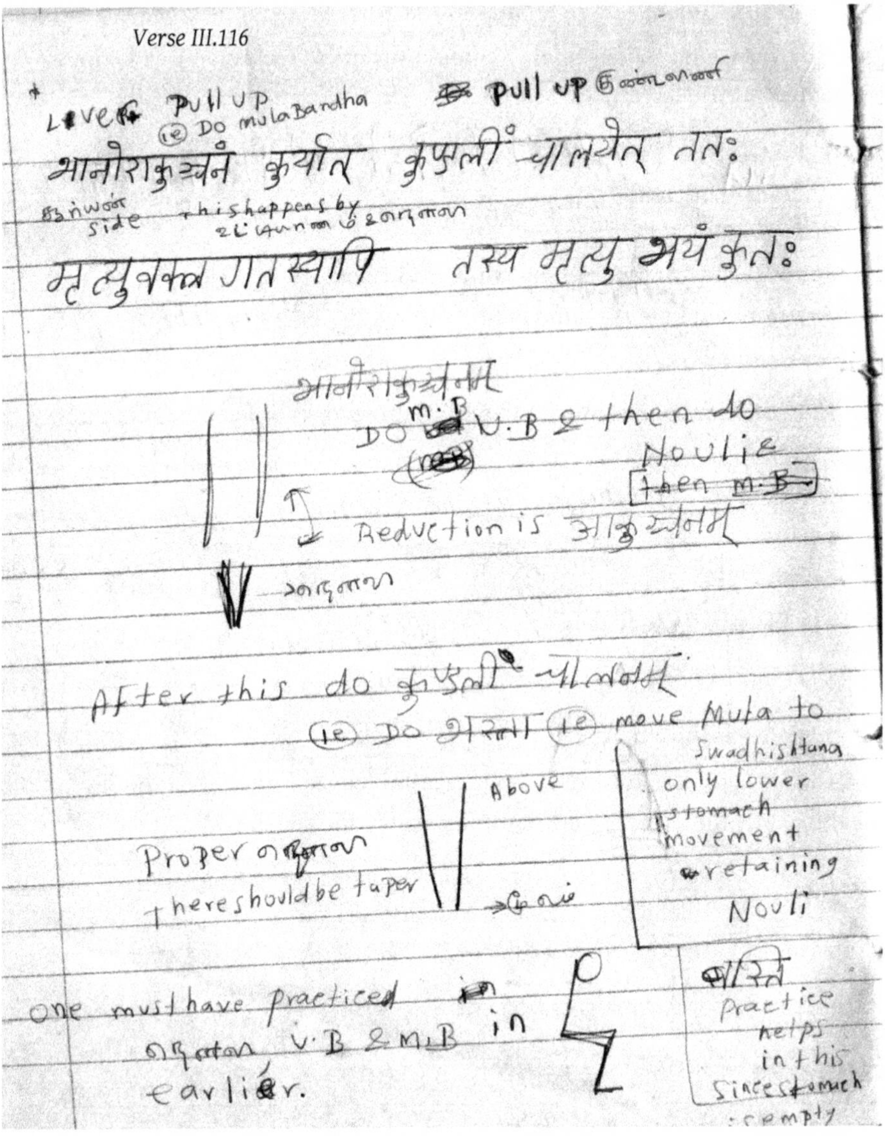

After this do bhastrikā (rapid inhale and exhale).

Then lift the mūlādhāra to svādhiṣṭhāna—lift the lower part of the pelvis and abdomen upward, while doing nauli.

To be successful in this, one must have first practiced nauli after uḍḍīyāna-bandha and mūla-bandha in ardha utkaṭāsana (chair pose).

Basti-kriyā (enema) can be useful to empty the colon and allow the abdomen to move without resistance.

Internally, the feeling of kuṇḍalinī arousal is like a muscle dissolving and mind becoming totally focused.

मुहूर्तद्वयपर्यन्तं निर्भयं चालनादसौ ।
ऊर्ध्वमाकृष्यते किञ्चित्सुषुम्नायां समुद्गता ॥११७॥

muhūrtadvayaparyantaṁ nirbhayaṁ cālanādasau |
ūrdhvamākṛṣyate kiñcitsuṣumnāyāṁ samudgatā ||117||

III.117: By moving [the kuṇḍalinī] without fear for about an hour and a half, she is drawn into the suṣumnā and moves upwards a little.

[Krishnamacharya] The text says, "without fear," because such prolonged practice can sometimes lead to bleeding.

तेन कुण्डलिनी तस्याः सुषुम्नाया मुखं ध्रुवम् ।
जहाति तस्मात्प्राणोऽयं सुषुम्नां व्रजति स्वतः ॥११८॥

tena kuṇḍalinī tasyāḥ suṣumnāyā mukhaṁ dhruvam |
jahāti tasmātprāṇo'yaṁ suṣumnāṁ vrajati svataḥ ||118||

III.118: Through this [process] the kuṇḍalinī leaves [open] the mouth of the suṣumnā and, therefore, prāṇa naturally enters the suṣumnā.

[Krishnamacharya] The method proposed in the previous verses is risky. Long inhalation and exhalation in headstand, with suspension of breath after exhalation for 10 seconds and longer can produce the same effect.

तस्मात्सञ्चालयेन्नित्यं सुखसुप्तामरुन्धतीम् ।
तस्याः सञ्चालनेनैव योगी रोगैः प्रमुच्यते ॥११९॥

tasmātsañcālayennityaṁ sukhasuptāmarundhatīm |
tasyāḥ sañcālanenaiva yogī rogaiḥ pramucyate ||119||

III.119: Therefore, one should daily move the kuṇḍalinī who is sleeping comfortably. Only by moving her, the yogi is freed from disease.

[Krishnamacharya] The text says that awakening or moving the kuṇḍalinī is the solution for all problems!

येन सञ्चालिता शक्तिः स योगी सिद्धिभाजनम् ।
किमत्र बहुनोक्तेन कालं जयति लीलया ॥१२०॥

yena sañcālitā śaktiḥ sa yogī siddhibhājanam |
kimatra bahunoktena kālaṁ jayati līlayā ||120||

III.120: The yogi who moves the śakti (kuṇḍalinī) becomes the possessor of the special powers (siddhi-s). What more need to be said? He conquers time (i.e. death) as if it were mere play.

ब्रह्मचर्यरतस्यैव नित्यं हितमिताशिनः ।
मण्डलाद्दृश्यते सिद्धिः कुण्डल्यभ्यासयोगिनः ॥१२१॥

brahmacaryaratasyaiva nityaṁ hitamitāśinaḥ |
maṇḍalāddṛśyate siddhiḥ kuṇḍalyabhyāsayoginaḥ ||121||

III.121: One who is dedicated to brahmacarya (celibacy), always following a healthy and moderate diet, and practicing yoga in the form of moving the kuṇḍalinī, will have success in forty days.

[Krishnamacharya] Note the contradiction here. The author suddenly says that brahmacarya is essential for awakening or moving the kuṇḍalinī but he advocated vajrolī a little earlier in this chapter!

कुण्डलीं चालयित्वा तु भस्त्रां कुर्याद्विशेषतः ।
एवमभ्यस्यतो नित्यं यमिनो यमभीः कुतः ॥१२२॥

kuṇḍalīṁ cālayitvā tu bhastrāṁ kuryādviśeṣataḥ |
evamabhyasyato nityaṁ yamino yamabhīḥ kutaḥ ||122||

III.122: Having moved the kuṇḍalinī, bhastrikā must be practiced carefully. Where is the fear of death for the self-restrained [yogi] who practices daily in this manner?

[Krishnamacharya] Proper Vedic chanting with ghana-pāṭha can give the same results.

द्वासप्ततिसहस्राणां नाडीनां मलशोधने ।
कुतः प्रक्षालनोपायः कुण्डल्यभ्यसनादृते ॥१२३॥

dvāsaptatisahasrāṇāṁ nāḍīnāṁ malaśodhane |
kutaḥ prakṣālanopāyaḥ kuṇḍalyabhyasanādṛte ||123||

III.123: Except the practice of [moving] the kuṇḍalinī [through śakti-cālana], what other means is there to cleanse the seventy-two thousand nāḍī-s of their impurities?

[Krishnamacharya] Viparītakaraṇī mudrā with long exhalation and suspension after exhalation can help to remove the impurities; kuṇḍalinī-cālana is not essential.

इयं तु मध्यमा नाडी दृढाभ्यासेन योगिनाम् ।
आसनप्राणसंयाममुद्राभिः सरला भवेत् ॥१२४॥

iyaṁ tu madhyamā nāḍī dṛḍhābhyāsena yogināṁ |
āsanaprāṇasaṁyāmamudrābhiḥ saralā bhavet ||124||

III.124: The central nāḍi (suṣumnā) is aligned [for the easy passage of prāṇa] in yogis persevering in the practice of āsana, prāṇāyāma, and mudrā-s.

[Krishnamacharya] By vajrāsana and bhastrikā, movement of the kuṇḍalinī can be achieved. Once it is moved or awakened, the serpent like shape becomes straight and flow of prāṇa happens through the central channel. For this, āsana, prāṇāyāma, and mudrā need to be practiced. So why is śakti-cālana essential?

अभ्यासे तु विनिद्राणां मनो धृत्वा समाधिना ।
रुद्राणी वा परा मुद्रा भद्रां सिद्धिं प्रयच्छति ॥१२५॥

abhyāse tu vinidrāṇāṁ mano dhṛtvā samādhinā |
rudrāṇī vā parā mudrā bhadrāṁ siddhiṁ prayacchati ||125||

III, 125: For those who are alert and free from indolence in practice, whose minds are steady in a state of focus, the rudrāṇī (śāṁbhavī) or other mudrā-s bestow great fulfilment.

[Krishnamacharya] The śāṁbhavī-mudrā mentioned here is the same as śanmukhī-mudrā of the Yoga Yājñavalkya (VI.50-53). Through ṣaṇmukhī-mudrā with vṛtti-nirodha (stillness of the mind), desired results can be attained without practicing kuṇḍalinī movement or awakening.

राजयोगं विना पृथ्वी राजयोगं विना निशा ।
राजयोगं विना मुद्रा विचित्रापि न शोभते ॥ १२६ ॥

rājayogaṁ vinā pṛthvī rājayogaṁ vinā niśā |
rājayogaṁ vinā mudrā vicitrāpi na śobhate ||126 ||

III.126: There is no earth without raja-yoga, there is no night without raja-yoga, and all the mudrā-s become useless without raja-yoga.

[Krishnamacharya] Without āsana and prāṇāyāma, there is no steadiness of mind.

Without good inhalation and exhalation, there is no prāṇāyāma.

Without controlled long inhalations and exhalations, mahāmudrā and śanmukhī-mudrā will not fructify.

While āsana and prāṇāyāma are included in rāja-yoga texts (e.g. Yoga Sūtra), śakti-cālana is a practice only in haṭha-yoga texts.

मारुतस्य विधिं सर्वं मनोयुक्तं समभ्यसेत् ।
इतरत्र न कर्तव्या मनोवृत्तिर्मनीषिणा ॥ १२७ ॥

mārutasya vidhiṁ sarvaṁ manoyuktaṁ samabhyaset |
itaratra na kartavyā manovṛttirmanīṣiṇā ||127 ||

III.127: All practices concerning breath [control] should be done with mindfulness. A wise person should not allow his mind to wander elsewhere.

[Krishnamacharya] Yoga Sūtra II.47 is referred to here: a balance of effort and relaxation is required.

इति मुद्रा दश प्रोक्ता आदिनाथेन शम्भुना ।
एकैका तासु यमिनां महासिद्धिप्रदायिनी ॥ १२८ ॥

iti mudrā daśa proktā ādināthena śambhunā |
ekaikā tāsu yamināṁ mahāsiddhipradāyinī ||128||

III.128: Thus, the ten mudrā-s have been described by Ādinātha who is [none other than] Lord Śiva. Each one of them bestows great powers on the self-restrained practitioners.

उपदेशं हि मुद्राणां यो दत्ते साम्प्रदायिकम् ।
स एव श्रीगुरुः स्वामी साक्षादीश्वर एव सः ॥१२९ ॥

upadeśaṁ hi mudrāṇāṁ yo datte sāmpradāyikam |
sa eva śrīguruḥ svāmī sākṣādīśvara eva saḥ ||129 ||

III.129: One who teaches the mudrā-s as handed down by the lineage of teachers is the guru. He is the master and the Lord (Īśvara) himself.

तस्य वाक्यपरो भूत्वा मुद्राभ्यासे समाहितः ।
अणिमादिगुणैः सार्धं लभते कालवञ्चनम् ॥१३० ॥

tasya vākyaparo bhūtvā mudrābhyāse samāhitaḥ |
aṇimādiguṇaiḥ sārdhaṁ labhate kālavañcanam ||130 ||

III.130: One who carefully follows his teachings, concentrating on the practice of the mudrā-s, attains various special powers and overcomes death.

[Krishnamacharya] In the Gheraṇḍa Saṁhitā, śakti-cālana is described thus:

Encircling the loins with a piece of cloth, seated in a secret room, let him practice śakti-cālana. One cubit long, and four fingers (i.e. 3 inches) wide, should be the encircling cloth, soft, white and of fine texture. Join this cloth with the kati-sūtra (i.e. a string worn round the loins.)

Rub the body with ashes, sit in the siddhāsana posture, draw the prāṇa-vāyu through the nostrils, and firmly join it with the apāna. Contract the rectum slowly by the aśvinī-mudrā, until the prāṇa enters the suṣumnā and manifests its presence.

Restraining the breath by kumbhaka in this way, the serpent kuṇḍalinī, feeling suffocated, awakes and rises upwards to the brahmarandhra.

Chapter IV

Chapter IV: Detailed Summary

1-2: Introduction

3-4: Synonyms of samādhi.

5-7: Three definitions of samādhi.

8-9: Praise of samādhi.

10-14: Moving or awakening the kuṇḍalinī and the result.

15-25: Relationship between mind and prāṇa.

25-30: Mind and vitality.

31-34: Definition and categories of laya.

35-42: Means for laya.

43-50: Khecarī mudrā and yoga-nidrā.

51-64: Non-dualism.

65-68: Nādānusandhāna (experiencing subtle inner sound or vibration).

69-77: The four stages of laya yoga, piercing the three cakra-s through the practice of prāṇāyāma and its result—rāja-yoga according to this text.

82-89: Nādānusandhāna and samādhi.

90-103: Nādānusandhāna illustrated through similes.

104-115: Praise.

Chapter IV: Translation

चतुर्थोपदेशः

caturthopadeśaḥ

नमः शिवाय गुरवे नादबिन्दुकलात्मने ।
निरञ्जनपदं याति नित्यं तत्र परायणः ॥ १ ॥

namaḥ śivāya gurave nādabindukalātmane |
nirañjanapadaṁ yāti nityaṁ tatra parāyaṇaḥ ||1||

IV.1: Salutations to Lord Śiva, the guru, who is in the form of nāda (audible and normally experienced sound), bindu (subtle sensation of sound), and kalā (the subtlest experience of sound, in the form of tanmātra, its origin). One who is devoted to these attains the state of freedom.

[Krishnamacharya] The word "Śiva" means "auspicious" and "peaceful." It can refer to one's own guru or the Divine.

अथेदानीं प्रवक्ष्यामि समाधिक्रममुत्तमम् ।
मृत्युघ्नं च सुखोपायं ब्रह्मानन्दकरं परम् ॥ २ ॥

athedānīṁ pravakṣyāmi samādhikramamuttamam |
mṛtyughnaṁ ca sukhopāyaṁ brahmānandakaraṁ param ||2||

IV.2: Now I shall expound the excellent process of attaining samādhi, which destroys death, leads to happiness, and confers supreme bliss in Brahman.

राजयोगः समाधिश्च उन्मनी च मनोन्मनी ।
अमरत्वं लयस्तत्त्वं शून्याशून्यं परं पदम् ॥ ३ ॥
अमनस्कं तथाद्वैतं निरालम्बं निरञ्जनम् ।
जीवन्मुक्तिश्च सहजा तुर्या चेत्येकवाचकाः ॥ ४ ॥

rājayogaḥ samādhiśca unmanī ca manonmanī |
amaratvaṁ layastattvaṁ śūnyāśūnyaṁ paraṁ padam ||3||

amanaskaṁ tathādvaitaṁ nirālambaṁ nirañjanam |
jīvanmuktiśca sahajā turyā cetyekavācakāḥ ||4||

IV.3-4: Rāja-yoga, samādhi, unmanī, manonmanī, amaratva (immortality), laya (absorption), tattva (truth), śūnyāśūnya (void and yet not void), paramapada (the supreme state), amanaska (transcending the mind), advaita (non-duality), nirālamba (without support), nirañjana (pure), jīvanmukti (liberation while in the body), sahaja (natural state) and turyā (transcendent or fourth state) are all synonyms.

[Krishnamacharya] These two verses propose numerous synonyms for samādhi (complete absorption of the mind). These words do not all mean the same; the text offers no definition of each and is imprecise in their usage. This can cause confusion as can be seen later in this chapter.

सलिले सैन्धवं यद्वत्साम्यं भजति योगतः ।
तथात्ममनसोरैक्यं समाधिरभिधीयते ॥५॥

salile saindhavaṁ yadvatsāmyaṁ bhajati yogataḥ |
tathātmamanasoraikyaṁ samādhirabhidhīyate ||5||

IV.5: Just as salt dissolves in water, the merging of mind and self (ātman) is called samādhi.

[Krishnamacharya] The point here is the dissolution of the latent impressions in the mind.

यदा संक्षीयते प्राणो मानसं च प्रलीयते ।
तदा समरसत्वं च समाधिरभिधीयते ॥६॥

yadā saṁkṣīyate prāṇo mānasaṁ ca pralīyate |
tadā samarasatvaṁ ca samādhirabhidhīyate ||6||

IV.6: When the prāṇa is restrained and the mind is absorbed [in the self], that state of harmony is called samādhi.

[Krishnamacharya] The concept of diminishment of the scattering of prāṇa is presented clearly in the Yoga Yājñavalkya as well. The Yoga Sūtra I.3 presents the absorption of the mind in the self.

तत्समं च द्वयोरैक्यं जीवात्मपरमात्मनोः ।
प्रनष्टसर्वसङ्कल्पः समाधिः सोऽभिधीयते ॥७॥

tatsamaṁ ca dvayoraikyaṁ jīvātmaparamātmanoḥ |
pranaṣṭasarvasaṅkalpaḥ samādhiḥ so'bhidhīyate ||7||

IV.7: The state of equilibrium which is the union of the individual consciousness (jīvātma) and universal or divine consciousness (paramātma), in which there is an end to all intentions, is called samādhi.

राजयोगस्य माहात्म्यं को वा जानाति तत्वतः ।
ज्ञानं मुक्तिः स्थितिः सिद्धिर्गुरुवाक्येन लभ्यते ॥८॥

rājayogasya māhātmyaṁ ko vā jānāti tatvataḥ |
jñānaṁ muktiḥ sthitiḥ siddhirguruvākyena labhyate ||8||

IV.8: Who really knows the greatness of rāja-yoga? Knowledge (jñāna), freedom (mukti), stability (sthiti), and success (siddhi) are attained through the teachings of the guru.

दुर्लभो विषयत्यागो दुर्लभं तत्त्वदर्शनम् ।
दुर्लभा सहजावस्था सदा गुरोः करुणां विना ॥९॥

durlabho viṣayatyāgo durlabhaṁ tattva-darśanam |
durlabhā sahajāvasthā sadā guroḥ karuṇāṁ vinā ||9||

IV.9: Without the compassion of a true teacher, the renunciation of sensual pleasures, the experience of reality (tattva), and the natural state of being (sahajāvasthā) are difficult to attain.

विविधैरासनैः कुंभैर्विचित्रैः करणैरपि ।
प्रबुद्धायां महाशक्तौ प्राणः शून्ये प्रलीयते ॥१०॥

vividhairāsanaiḥ kuṁbhairvicitraiḥ karaṇairapi |
prabuddhāyāṁ mahāśaktau prāṇaḥ śūnye pralīyate ||10||

IV.10: When the great power (kuṇḍalinī) has been awakened by various āsana-s, prāṇāyāma-s, and mudrā-s, the prāṇa is absorbed in the void (i.e. brahmarandhra).

उत्पन्नशक्तिबोधस्य त्यक्तनिःशेषकर्मणः ।
योगिनः सहजावस्था स्वयमेव प्रजायते ॥११॥

utpannaśaktibodhasya tyaktaniḥśeṣakarmaṇaḥ |
yoginaḥ sahajāvasthā svayameva prajāyate ||11||

IV.11: In the yogi in whom the energy (kuṇḍalinī) is awakened, and who has relinquished all actions, the natural state (sahajāvasthā) comes into being on its own.

[Krishnamacharya] When the mind becomes steady by prāṇa entering suṣumnā, the natural state or experience of self is attained. As noted earlier, this is the state referred to in Yoga Sūtra I.3.

सुषुम्नावाहिनि प्राणे शून्ये विशति मानसे ।
तदा सर्वाणि कर्माणि निर्मूलयति योगवित् ॥ १२ ॥

suṣumnāvāhini prāṇe śūnye viśati mānase |
tadā sarvāṇi karmāṇi nirmūlayati yogavit ||12||

IV.12: When prāṇa flows into suṣumnā and the mind is absorbed in the void, the knower of yoga uproots all his actions.

अमराय नमस्तुभ्यं सोऽपि कालस्त्वया जितः ।
पतितं वदने यस्य जगदेतच्चराचरम् ॥ १३ ॥

amarāya namastubhyaṁ so'pi kālastvayā jitaḥ |
patitaṁ vadane yasya jagadetaccarācaram ||13||

IV.13: Salutations to the immortal [yogi] who has conquered even time, into whose jaws has fallen this universe, with all its animate beings and inanimate objects.

चित्ते समत्वमापन्ने वायौ व्रजति मध्यमे ।
तदामरोली वज्रोली सहजोली प्रजायते ॥ १४ ॥

citte samatvamāpanne vāyau vrajati madhyame |
tadāmarolī vajrolī sahajolī prajāyate ||14||

IV.14: When the mind has reached a state of equanimity, and prāṇa moves through the center [nāḍī] (suṣumnā), then amarolī, vajrolī, and sahajolī manifest on their own.

[Krishnamacharya] The text says here that when the mind becomes steady, prāṇa goes into the suṣumnā, and this leads automatically to success in vajrolī, sahajolī, and amarolī. If this is the case, then where is the need to practice vajrolī, sahajolī, or amarolī?

ज्ञानं कुतो मनसि सम्भवतीह तावत्
प्राणोऽपि जीवति मनो म्रियते न यावत् ।
प्राणो मनो द्वयमिदं विलयं नयेद्यो
मोक्षं स गच्छति नरो न कथंचिदन्यः ॥ १५ ॥

jñānaṁ kuto manasi sambhavatīha tāvat
prāṇo'pi jīvati mano mriyate na yāvat |
prāṇo mano dvayamidaṁ vilayaṁ nayedyo
mokṣaṁ sa gacchati naro na kathaṁcidanyaḥ ||15||

IV.15: Experience [of the self] cannot be attained so long as the prāṇa is scattered and the mind is active (i.e. restless). Only the one who quietens the mind and prāṇa attains liberation.

ज्ञात्वा सुषुम्नासद्भेदं कृत्वा वायुं च मध्यगम् ।
स्थित्वा सदैव सुस्थाने ब्रह्मरन्ध्रे निरोधयेत् ॥ १६ ॥

jñātvā suṣumṇāsadbhedaṁ kṛtvā vāyuṁ ca madhyagam |
sthitvā sadaiva susthāne brahmarandhre nirodhayet ||16||

IV.16: Knowing well to open the suṣumnā, and [then] making the prāṇa flow through the center [nāḍī], it should be restrained, in a sound place, in the crown of the head (brahmarandhra).

[Krishnamacharya] "In a sound place" here refers to the crown of the head where the prāṇa is channeled, not to where the yogi physically resides.

सूर्यचन्द्रमसौ धत्तः कालं रात्रिन्दिवात्मकम् ।
भोक्त्री सुषुम्ना कालस्य गुह्यमेतदुदाहृतम् ॥ १७ ॥

sūryacandramasau dhattaḥ kālaṁ rātrindivātmakam |
bhoktrī suṣumnā kālasya guhyametadudāhṛtam ||17||

IV.17: The sun and the moon create [the division of] time in the form of day and night. Suṣumnā consumes time; this is said to be a secret.

[Krishnamacharya] The sun and moon are markers of external time. Similarly, the movement of prāṇa in the two channels of iḍā and piṅgalā create the inner experience of time. When prāṇa is in suṣumnā, the yogi does not experience the passage of time.

द्वासप्ततिसहस्राणि नाडीद्वाराणि पञ्जरे ।
सुषुम्ना शाम्भवी शक्तिः शेषास्त्वेव निरर्थकाः ॥१८॥

dvāsaptatisahasrāṇi nāḍīdvārāṇi pañjare |
suṣumnā śāmbhavī śaktiḥ śeṣāstveva nirarthakāḥ ||18||

IV.18: There are 72,000 nāḍi-s in this cage (i.e. the body). Of these, suṣumnā or śāmbhavī is the one with power. The other nāḍi-s are not of much use.

[Krishnamacharya] Such praise is excessive and unnecessary (sphīta-doṣa).

वायुः परिचितो यस्मादग्निना सह कुण्डलीम् ।
बोधयित्वा सुषुम्नायां प्रविशेदनिरोधतः ॥१९॥

vāyuḥ paricito yasmādagninā saha kuṇḍalīm |
bodhayitvā suṣumnāyāṁ praviśedanirodhataḥ ||19||

IV.19: When breath is controlled, it arouses the kuṇḍalinī along with the metabolic fire and enters the suṣumnā without any restriction.

[Krishnamacharya] Agni along with prāṇa enter suṣumnā as noted in the Yoga Yājñavalkya. Kuṇḍalinī is explained more clearly in Yoga Yājñavalkya than in the Haṭha Yoga Pradīpikā.

सुशुम्नावाहिनि प्राणे सिद्ध्यत्येव मनोन्मनी ।
अन्यथा त्वितराभ्यासाः प्रयासयैव योगिनाम् ॥२०॥

suśumnāvāhini prāṇe siddhyatyeva manonmanī |
anyathā tvitarābhyāsāḥ prayāsayaiva yoginām ||20||

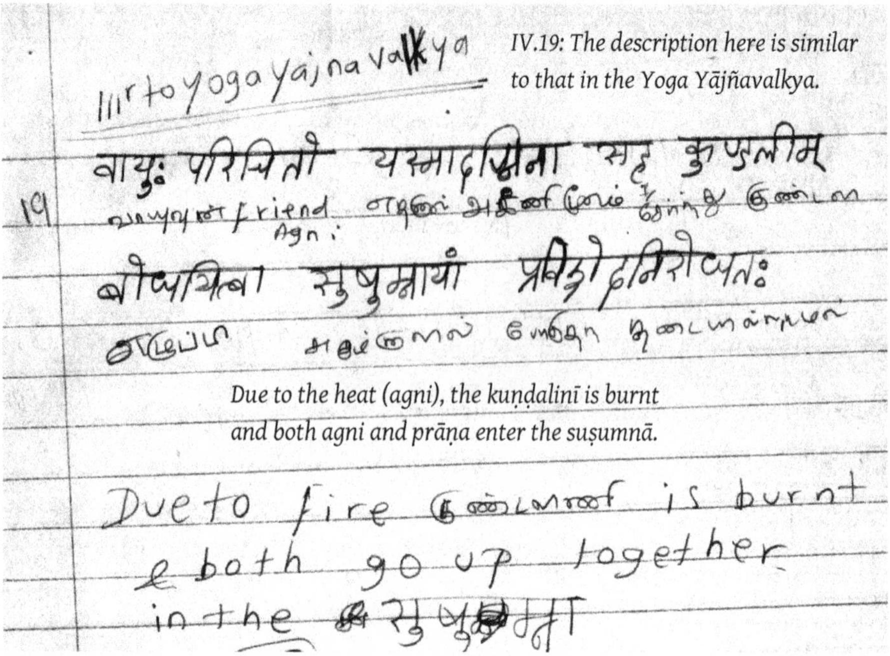

IV.19: The description here is similar to that in the Yoga Yājñavalkya.

Due to the heat (agni), the kuṇḍalinī is burnt and both agni and prāṇa enter the suṣumnā.

IV.20: When prāṇā flows through suṣumnā, the manonmanī (i.e. samādhi) state is attained. Without this, the other practices are mere exertion for the yogi.

[Krishnamacharya] This is excessive praise.

पवनो बध्यते येन मनस्तेनैव बध्यते ।

मनश्च बध्यते येन पवनस्तेन बध्यते ॥२१॥

pavano badhyate yena manastenaiva badhyate |
manaśca badhyate yena pavanastena badhyate ||21||

IV.21: One who controls the breath controls the mind. One who controls the mind controls the breath.

हेतुद्वयं तु चित्तस्य वासना च समीरणः ।

तयोर्विनष्ट एकस्मिन् तौ द्वावपि विनश्यतः ॥२२॥

hetudvayaṁ tu cittasya vāsanā ca samīraṇaḥ |
tayorvinaṣṭa ekasmin tau dvāvapi vinaśyataḥ ||22||

IV.22: The activity of the mind is based on two factors: prāṇa and the latent impressions (vāsanā). When one of these becomes inactive the other also comes to an end.

[Krishnamacharya] This verse is not entirely correct, and the same idea is extended in subsequent verses too. When prāṇa subsides, the mind will also subside. But that does not mean that the latent impressions or saṁskāra-s in the mind have reduced. Appropriate meditation (dhyāna) is essential to change the saṁskāra-s.

मनो यत्र विलीयेत पवनस्तत्र लीयते ।
पवनो लीयते यत्र मनस्तत्र विलीयते ॥२३॥

mano yatra vilīyeta pavanastatra līyate |
pavano līyate yatra manastatra vilīyate ||23||

IV.23: Where the mind is absorbed, there the prāṇa is absorbed. Where the prāṇa is absorbed, there the mind is absorbed.

दुग्धाम्बुवत्संमिलितावुभौ तौ तुल्यक्रियौ मानसमारुतौ हि ।
यतो मरुत्तत्र मनःप्रवृत्तिर्यतो मनस्तत्र मरुतप्रवृत्तिः ॥२४॥

dugdhāmbuvatsaṁmilitāvubhau tau tulyakriyau mānasamārutau hi |
yato maruttatra manaḥpravṛttiryato manastatra marutapravṛttiḥ ||24||

IV.24: When mind and prāṇa are mingled like milk and water, their activities coincide (tulya-kriyā). Where the breath (prāṇa) is active, there the mind is [also active]. Where there is activity of the mind, there the breath (prāṇa) is [also active].

तत्रैकनाशादपरस्य नाश एकप्रवृत्तेरपरप्रवृत्तिः ।
अध्वस्तयोश्चयोश्चेन्द्रियवर्गवृत्तिः प्रध्वस्तयोर्मोक्षपदस्य सिद्धिः ॥२५॥

tatraikanāśādaparasya nāśa ekapravṝtteraparapravṝttiḥ |
adhvastayośendriyavargavṝttiḥ pradhvastayormokṣhapadasya siddhiḥ ||25||

IV.25: If one is destroyed, the other is set at rest. The action of one leads to the action of the other. If both are not quietened, the senses remain active. If they are controlled, the state of liberation is attained.

रसस्य मनसश्चैव चञ्चलत्वं सवभावतः ।
रसो बद्धो मनो बद्धं किं न सिद्ध्यति भूतले ॥२६॥

rasasya manasaścaiva cañcalatvaṁ svabhāvataḥ |
raso baddho mano baddhaṁ kiṁ na siddhyati bhūtale ||26||

IV.26: Mercury and mind are both unsteady by nature. If mercury can be stabilized, the mind can also be steadied. What then is impossible to attain on this earth?

मूर्च्छितो हरते व्याधीन् मृतो जीवयति स्वयम् ।
बद्धः खेछरतां धत्ते रसो वायुश्च पार्वति ॥२७॥

mūrcchito harate vyādhīn mṛto jīvayati svayam |
baddhaḥ khecaratāṁ dhatte raso vāyuśca pārvati ||27||

IV.27: O Pārvati! When [mind and mercury] are made inactive they destroy diseases. They also lead to longevity. When they are bound, they give rise to success in khecarī.

मनः स्थैर्ये स्थिरो वायुस्ततो बिन्दुः स्थिरो भवेत् ।
बिन्दुस्थैर्यात् सदा सत्त्वं पिण्डस्थैर्यं प्रजायते ॥२८॥

manaḥ sthairye sthiro vāyustato binduḥ sthiro bhavet |
bindusthairyāt sadā sattvaṁ piṇḍasthairyaṁ prajāyate ||28||

IV.28: When the mind is steady, the prāṇa is steady and therefore there is stability of vitality (i.e. sexual urge). When vitality is stable, it brings about strength which manifests in the body.

[Krishnamacharya] Vitality (amṛta-bindu) referred to here is related to Yoga Sūtra II.38 on the practice of control over the urge for sex. The pulse is also related to steadiness of the mind. Through the practice of yoga, with control over the mind, the pulse should reduce to as low as forty-five per minute. There are two Upaniṣats on these topics. The Amṛta Bindu Upaniṣat deals with preservation of vitality and Nāda Bindu Upaniṣat deals with inner sound. Preservation of vitality is essential for hearing the inner sound.

इन्द्रियाणां मनो नाथो मनोनाथस्तु मारुतः ।
मारुतस्य लयो नाथः स लयो नादमाश्रितः ॥२९॥

indriyāṇāṁ mano nātho manonāthastu mārutaḥ |
mārutasya layo nāthaḥ sa layo nādamāśritaḥ ||29||

IV.29: Mind is the master of the senses. Prāṇa is the master of the mind. Absorption (laya) is the master of prāṇa and, absorption is dependent on inner sound (nāda).

सोऽयमेवास्तु मोक्षाख्यो मास्तु वापि मतान्तरे ।
मनःप्राणलये कश्चिदानन्दः संप्रवर्तते ॥३०॥

so'yamevāstu mokṣākhyo māstu vāpi matāntare |
manaḥprāṇalaye kaścidānandaḥ saṁpravartate ||30||

IV.30: When the prāṇa and mind are in a state of absorption, an indefinable bliss ensues. This itself can be called liberation. Some may not agree with this.

[Krishnamacharya] One pointed focus of the mind arises from this practice, not mokṣa or liberation.

प्रनष्टश्वासनिश्वासः प्रध्वस्तविषयग्रहः ।
निश्चेष्टो निर्विकारश्च लयो जयति योगिनाम् ॥३१॥

pranaṣṭaśvāsaniśvāsaḥ pradhvastaviṣayagrahaḥ |
niśceṣṭo nirvikāraśca layo jayati yoginām ||31||

IV.31: When inhalation and exhalation are suspended, when the senses cease to grasp objects, when there is no movement in the body, and no activities in the mind, the yogi has succeeded in absorption.

[Krishnamacharya] Here the section on laya-yoga begins. The laya-yogi is one whose prāṇa is in suṣumnā.

उच्छिन्नसर्वसंकल्पो निःशेषाशेषचेष्टितः ।
स्वावगम्यो लयः कोऽपि जायते वागगोचरः ॥३२॥

ucchinnasarvasaṁkalpo niḥśeṣāśeṣaceṣṭitaḥ |
svāvagamyo layaḥ ko'pi jāyate vāgagocaraḥ ||32||

IV.32: When all mental activities completely cease, when there is no physical movement, a state of absorption ensues, which can be understood only by oneself and is beyond the reach of words.

[Krishnamacharya] This place of laya is the anāhata-cakra. Speech dissolves in mind, mind in prāṇa, prāṇa in the individual self, and the self in the Divine.

यत्र दृष्टिर्लयस्तत्र भूतेन्द्रियसनातनी ।
सा शक्तिर्जीवभूतानां द्वे अलक्ष्ये लयं गते ॥३३॥

yatra dṛṣṭirlayastatra bhūtendriyasanātanī |
sā śaktirjīvabhūtānāṁ dve alakṣye layaṁ gate ||33||

IV.33: Where focus is [directed] there [in Brahman], one becomes absorbed. That by which the five elements and the senses exist, and the energy (śakti) of all living beings—both are dissolved in the characterless [Brahman].

[Krishnamacharya] In the state of laya, there is neither vidyā nor avidyā.

लयो लय इति प्राहुः कीदृशं लयलक्षणम् ।
अपुनर्वासनोत्थानाल्लयो विषयविस्मृतिः ॥३४॥

layo laya iti prāhuḥ kīdṛśaṁ layalakṣaṇam |
apunarvāsanotthānāllayo viṣayavismṛtiḥ ||34||

IV.34: People say 'laya, laya!' but what is the nature of laya? Laya is not recollecting the objects of the senses, since latent impressions (vāsanā-s) do not recur.

[Krishnamacharya] Laya is when prāṇa is arrested in suṣumnā. Laya is defined as absence of perception. The author claims vāsanā-s will not arise again, but this is not true.

वेदशास्त्रपुराणानि सामान्यगणिका इव ।
एकैव शांभवी मुद्रा गुप्ता कुलवधूरिव ॥३५॥

vedaśāstrapurāṇāni sāmānyagaṇikā iva |
ekaiva śāṁbhavī mudrā guptā kulavadhūriva ||35||

IV.35: The Vedas, śastra-s (traditional texts), and purāṅa-s (traditional stories) are like common courtesans. But the śāṁbhavī-mudrā is guarded like a noble woman.

[Krishnamacharya] Excessive and unnecessary praise again (sphīta-doṣa).

अन्तर्लक्ष्यं बहिर्दृष्टिर्निमेषोन्मेषवर्जिता ।
एषा सा शांभवी मुद्रा वेदशास्त्रेषु गोपिता ॥३६॥

antarlakṣyaṁ bahirdṛṣṭirnimeṣonmeṣavarjitā |
eṣā sā śāṁbhavī mudrā vedaśāstreṣu gopitā ||36||

IV.36: Concentrating inwards, with open eyes and without blinking, is śāṁbhavī-mudrā, which is preserved in the Vedas and śāstra-s.

[Krishnamacharya] The author contradicts himself between this verse and the previous one. While the previous verse claims that this mudrā is special and different from what is in the Vedas and related texts, this verse says the opposite.

अन्तर्लक्ष्यविलीनचित्तपवनो योगी यदा वर्तते
दृष्ट्या निश्चलतारया बहिरधः पश्यन्नपश्यन्नपि ।
मुद्रेयं खलु शांभवी भवति सा लब्धा प्रसादाद् गुरोः
शून्याशून्यविलक्षणं स्फुरति तत् तत्त्वं पदं शांभवम् ॥३७॥

antarlakṣyavilīnacittapavano yogī yadā vartate
dṛṣṭayā niścalatārayā bahiradhaḥ paśyannapaśyannapi |
mudreyaṁ khalu śāṁbhavī bhavati sā labdhā prasādād guroḥ
śūnyāśūnyavilakṣaṇaṁ sfurati tat tattvaṁ padaṁ śāṁbhavam ||37||

IV.37: When the yogi remains with mind and breath absorbed in an internal object, his pupils motionless, his eyes without perceiving external objects, then it is indeed śāṁbhavī-mudrā. When obtained by the grace of the guru, that state which is of Śambhu (Śiva), which is apart from that which is manifest and non-manifest, that is experienced [by the yogi].

[Krishnamacharya] When the mind is stilled, automatically, prāṇa is stilled. One means to that is the practice of ṣaṇmukhī-mudrā. An alternative practice, based on light, is presented in the Śvetāśvatara Upaniṣat.

श्रीशांभव्याश्च खेचर्या अवस्थाधामभेदतः ।
भवेच्चित्तलयानन्दः शून्ये चित्सुखरूपिणि ॥३८॥

śrīśāṁbhavyāśca khecaryā avasthādhāmabhedataḥ |
bhaveccittalayānandaḥ śūnye citsukharūpiṇi ||38||

IV.38: The śāṁbhavī [mudrā] and the khecarī [mudrā] although differing in the focus of the eyes and the place [where the attention of the mind is directed], both bring about the bliss of absorption of the mind in the void (i.e. ātman or self) whose nature is bliss.

[Krishnamacharya] The place of focus in the śāṁbhavī-mudrā is the anāhata (heart center) and in khecarī mudrā it is the kaphāla-kuhara (space behind the palate). There is a book called Citsukhī related to non-dualism or advaita; this verse could be referring to that text. Refer Yoga Sūtra III.12 on ekāgratā-pariṇāma as well.

तारे ज्योतिषि संयोज्य किंचिदुन्नमयेद्भ्रुवौ ।
पूर्वयोगं मनो युञ्जन्नुन्मनीकारकः क्षणात् ॥३९॥

tāre jyotiṣi saṁyojya kiṁcidunnamayed bhruvau |
pūrvayogaṁ mano yuñjannunmanīkārakaḥ kṣaṇāt ||39||

IV.39: Directing the gaze towards the light [that arises when concentrating on the tip of the nose,] raise the eyebrows slightly. Concentrate the mind according to the previous practice, and absorption (unmanī) is quickly attained.

[Krishnamacharya] Steadiness of the gaze is related to steadiness of the mind. One method of increasing mental steadiness is through steadying the eyes.

केचिदागमजालेन केचिन्निगमसंकुलैः ।
केचित् तर्केण मुह्यन्ति नैव जानन्ति तारकम् ॥४०॥

kecidāgamajālena kecinnigamasaṁkulaiḥ |
kecit tarkeṇa muhyanti naiva jānanti tārakam ||40||

IV.40: Some are confused by the Vedas, some by tantra, and others by logic (tarka). They do not know tāraka (i.e. the state of unmanī).

[Krishnamacharya] Excessive praise again. The word tāraka here could also mean the praṇava ("OM"), that which helps to cross the ocean of life.

अर्धोन्मीलितलोचनः स्थिरमना नासाग्रदत्तेक्षण
श्चन्द्रार्कावपि लीनतामुपनयन्निस्पन्दभावेन यः ।
ज्योतीरूपमशेषबीजमखिलं देदीप्यमानं परं
तत्त्वं तत्पदमेति वस्तु परमं वाच्यं किमत्राधिकम् ॥४१॥

ardhonmīlitalocanaḥ sthiramanā nāsāgradattekṣaṇa
ścandrārkāvapi līnatāmupanayannispandabhāvena yaḥ |
jyotīrūpamaśeṣabījamakhilaṁ dedīpyamānaṁ paraṁ
tattvaṁ tatpadameti vastu paramaṁ vācyaṁ kimatrādhikam ||41||

IV.41: With half-closed eyes and steady mind, with the gaze directed to the tip of the nose, the one in whom the moon (iḍā or left side) and sun (piṅgalā or right side) are suspended, who is in a motionless state, he attains that abode which is resplendent light, the supreme reality and the source of all. What more needs to be said?

दिवा न पूजयेल्लिङ्गं रात्रौ चैव न पूजयेत् ।
सर्वदा पूजयेल्लिङ्गं दिवारात्रिनिरोधतः ॥४२॥

divā na pūjayelliṅgaṁ rātrau caiva na pūjayet |
sarvadā pūjayelliṅgaṁ divārātrinirodhataḥ ||42||

IV.42: Do not worship the self (liṅga) by day. Do not worship it at night. Restraining the night and day, the self should always be worshipped.

अथ खेचरी
सव्यदक्षिणनाडीस्थो मध्ये चरति मारुतः ।
तिष्ठते खेचरी मुद्रा तस्मिन् स्थाने न संशयः ॥४३॥

atha khecarī
savyadakṣiṇanāḍīstho madhye carati mārutaḥ |
tiṣṭhate khecarī mudrā tasmin sthāne na saṁśayaḥ ||43

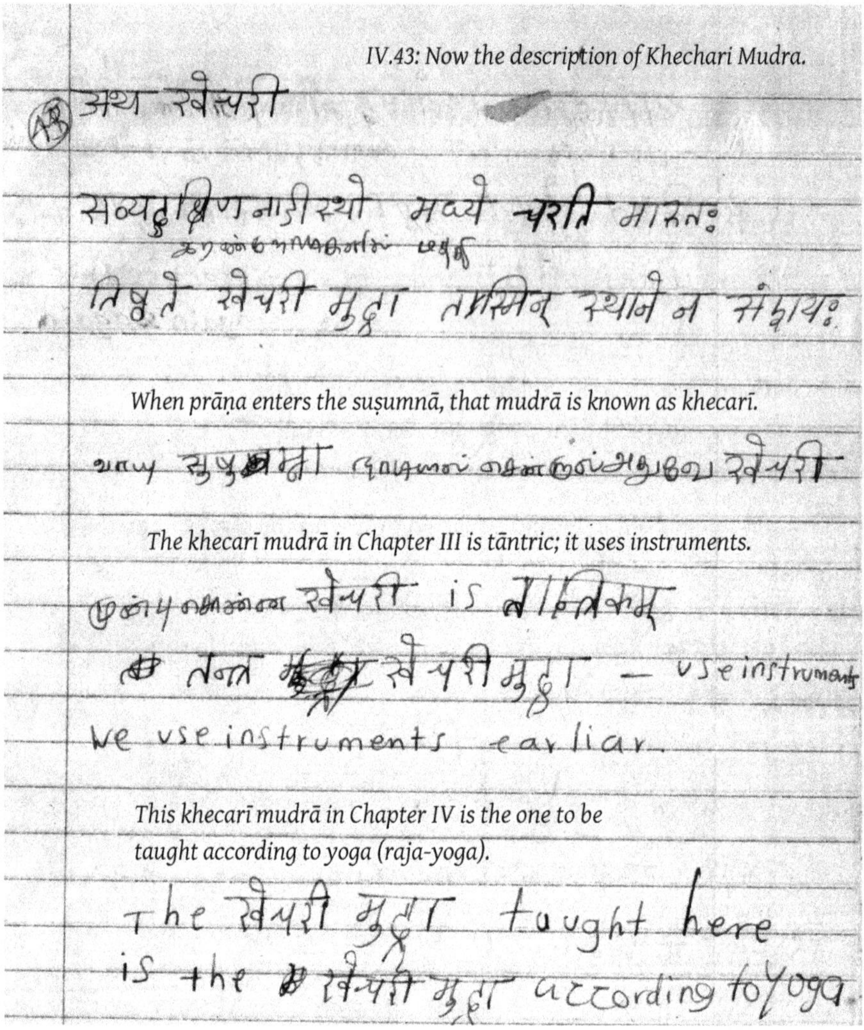

IV.43: Now the description of Khechari Mudra.

43 अथ खेचरी

सव्यदक्षिण नाडीस्थो मध्ये चरति मारुतः

तिष्ठते खेचरी मुद्रा तस्मिन् स्थाने न संशयः

When prāṇa enters the suṣumnā, that mudrā is known as khecarī.

The khecarī mudrā in Chapter III is tāntric; it uses instruments.

तन्त्र खेचरी मुद्रा — use instruments

we use instruments earliar.

This khecarī mudrā in Chapter IV is the one to be taught according to yoga (raja-yoga).

The खेचरी मुद्रा taught here is the खेचरी मुद्रा according to Yoga.

Now khecarī [mudrā is described]:

IV.43: When the prāṇa, which is in the left (iḍā) and right (piṅgalā) nāḍī-s, flows through the middle (suṣumnā), khecarī becomes firmly established. There is no doubt about this.

[Krishnamacharya] When the prāṇa enters suṣumnā, this is called khecarī.

इडापिङ्गलयोर्मध्ये शून्यं चैवानिलं ग्रसेत् ।
तिष्ठते खेचरी मुद्रा तत्र सत्यं पूनः पूनः ॥४४॥

iḍāpiṅgalayormadhye śūnyaṁ caivānilaṁ graset |
tiṣṭhate khecarī mudrā tatra satyaṁ pūnaḥ pūnaḥ ||44||

IV.44: When the void (śūnya) between the iḍā and piṅgalā swallows up the prāṇa (i.e. when prāṇa moves into suṣumnā), khecarī is firmly established. Practice it again and again.

सूर्याचन्द्रमसोर्मध्ये निरालम्बान्तरे पूनः ।
संस्थिता व्योमचक्रे या सा मुद्रा नाम खेचरी ॥४५॥

sūryācandramasormadhye nirālambāntare pūnaḥ |
saṁsthitā vyomacakre yā sā mudrā nāma khecarī ||45||

IV.45: Between the sun (piṅgalā) and moon (iḍā), in the unsupported space, in the space cakra, the mudrā that is practiced is called khecarī.

[Krishnamacharya] When the prāṇa enters the kaphāla-kuhara (space behind the palate), it is called khecarī in this Chapter IV. If the tongue presses into that same space, it is khecarī of the Chapter III.

सोमाद् यत्रोदिता धारा साक्षात् सा शिववल्लभा ।
पूरयेदतुलां दिव्यां सुषुम्नां पश्चिमे मुखे ॥४६॥

somād yatroditā dhārā sākṣāt sā śivavallabhāa |
pūrayedatulāṁ divyāṁ suṣumnāṁ paścime mukhe ||46||

IV.46: The stream of nectar flowing from the moon [through the practice of khecarī mudrā] is the place of Śiva. The mouth of the unequalled divine suṣumnā must be filled with it.

पुरस्ताच्चैव पूर्येत निश्चिता खेचरी भवेत् ।
अभ्यस्ता खेचरी मुद्राप्युन्मनी संप्रजायते ॥४७॥

purastāccaiva pūryeta niścitā khecarī bhavet |
abhyastā khecarī mudrāpyunmanī saṁprajāyate ||47||

IV.47: The mouth of the suṣumnā should also be filled from the front [through suspension of prāṇa]; that is the real khecarī. By the practice of khecarī mudrā the state of absorption (unmanī) is attained.

[Krishnamacharya] A particular type of prāṇāyāma known as vairambha prāṇāyāma is useful in this practice of khecarī mudrā.

भ्रुवोर्मध्ये शिवस्थानं मनस्तत्र विलीयते ।
ज्ञातव्यं तत्पदं तुर्यं तत्र कालो न विद्यते ॥४८ ॥

bhruvormadhye śivasthānaṁ manastatra vilīyate |
jñātavyaṁ tatpadaṁ turyaṁ tatra kālo na vidyate ||48||

IV.48: Between the eyebrows is the seat of Śiva, where the mind is in a state of absorption. This state is known as transcendent (turyā). In this state, one becomes unaware of time.

[Krishnamacharya] By proper meditation in that space, the mind quietens and is absorbed. In that state, as per this text, the mind is in the place of Śiva.

अभ्यसेत् खेचरीं तावद् यावत् स्याद् योगनिद्रितः ।
सम्प्राप्तयोगनिद्रस्य कालो नास्ति कदाचन ॥४९॥

abhyaset khecarīṁ tāvad yāvat syād yoganidritaḥ |
samprāptayoganidrasya kālo nāsti kadācana ||49||

IV.49: One should practice khecarī until yogic sleep (yoga-nidrā) is attained. For one who is in yogic sleep, there is no time.

[Krishnamacharya] Through the practice of the khecarī mudrā, yogic sleep (yoga-nidrā) comes about. Yogic sleep can also be understood to be restful and balanced (sattva-dominant) sleep. It is short, lasting only about three hours.

Yoga Sūtra defines sleep (nidrā) in I.10. Sleep is tamas-dominated in nature. Yogic sleep is not the same as the meditative absorption states (samādhi-s) of the Yoga Sūtra.

निरालम्बं मनः कृत्वा न किञ्चिदपि चिन्तयेत् ।
सबाह्याभ्यन्तरे व्योम्नि घटवत् तिष्ठति ध्रुवम् ॥५०॥

nirālambaṁ manaḥ kṛtvā na kiñcidapi cintayet |
sabāhyābhyantare vyomni ghaṭavat tiṣṭhati dhruvam ||50||

IV.50: After making the mind unsupported (i.e. freeing it of objects and concepts) one should not think of anything. He then remains like a pot filled inside and outside with space.

[Krishnamacharya] In the verses IV.51-64 to follow, the text makes a mixed presentation of concepts from non-dualism and Buddhism along with yoga philosophy. Krishnamacharya pointed out some of the flaws and contradictions in this presentation. Given the imprecise nature of the presentation in the original text, it is unnecessary to go into these details.

बाह्यवायुर्यथा लीनस्तथा मध्यो न संशयः ।
स्वस्थाने स्थिरतामेति पवनो मनसा सह ॥५१॥

bāhyavāyuryathā līnastathā madhyo na saṁśayaḥ |
svasthāne sthiratāmeti pavano manasā saha ||51||

IV.51: When the external breath is suspended [by the practice of khecarī], the breath inside is also suspended. There is no doubt about this. Then the prāṇa, along with the mind, becomes still in its own place.

एवमभ्यस्यतस्तस्य वायुमार्गे दिवानिशम् ।
अभ्यासाज्जीर्यते वायुर्मनस्तत्रैव लीयते ॥५२॥

evamabhyasyatastasya vāyumārge divāniśam |
abhyāsājjīryate vāyurmanastatraiva līyate ||52||

IV.52: In the practitioner who practices thus, channeling the prāṇa in its course [through the suṣumnā] night and day, where the prāṇa is absorbed through practice, there the mind is also absorbed.

अमृतैः प्लावयेद् देहमापादतलमस्तकम् ।
सिद्ध्यत्येव महाकायो महाबलपराक्रमः ॥५३॥

amṛtaiḥ plāvayed dehamāpādatalamastakam |
siddhyatyeva mahākāyo mahābalaparākramaḥ ||53||

IV.53: One should inundate the body from head to foot with the nectar [flowing from the moon]. This bestows [upon the yogi] a superior body, great strength, and valour. Thus, khecarī [has been described].

शक्तिमध्ये मनः कृत्वा शक्तिं मानसमध्यगाम् ।
मनसा मन आलोक्य धारयेत् परमं पदम् ॥५४॥

śaktimadhye manaḥ kṛtvā śaktiṁ mānasamadhyagām |
manasā mana ālokya dhārayet paramaṁ padam ||54||

IV.54: Centering the mind on the śakti (kuṇḍalinī), and the śakti in the center of the mind, observe the mind with the mind and meditate on the supreme state.

खमध्ये कुरु चात्मानमात्ममध्ये च खं कुरु ।
सर्वं च खमयं कृत्वा न किंचिदपि चिन्तयेत् ॥५५॥

khamadhye kuru cātmānamātmamadhye ca khaṁ kuru |
sarvaṁ ca khamayaṁ kṛtvā na kiṁcidapi cintayet ||55||

IV.55: Place the self (ātman) in the middle of space (ākāśa) and space in the midst of the self. Reducing everything to the nature of space, think of nothing else.

अन्तः शून्यो बहिः शून्यः शून्यः कुम्भ इवाम्बरे ।
अन्तः पूर्णो बहिः पूर्णः पूर्णः कुम्भ इवार्णवे ॥५६॥

antaḥ śūnyo bahiḥ śūnyaḥ śūnyaḥ kumbha ivāmbare |
antaḥ pūrṇo bahiḥ pūrṇaḥ pūrṇaḥ kumbha ivārṇave ||56||

IV.56: Void within, void without, void like a pot in space. Full inside, full outside, full like a pot in the ocean. [Such is the state of the yogi in this meditation.]

बाह्यचिन्ता न कर्तव्या तथैवान्तरचिन्तनम् ।
सर्वचिन्तां परित्यज्य न किंचिदपि चिन्तयेत् ॥५७॥

bāhyacintā na kartavyā tathaivāntaracintanam |
sarvacintāṁ parityajya na kiṁcidapi cintayet ||57||

IV.57: There should be no thought about external things or any thought about internal things. Relinquishing all such thoughts, [the yogi] should think of nothing.

संकल्पमात्रकलनैव जगत् समग्रं
संकल्पमात्रकलनैव मनोविलासः ।
संकल्पमात्रमतिमुत्सृज निर्विकल्पम्
आश्रित्य निश्चयमवाप्नुहि राम शान्तिम् ॥५८॥

saṁkalpamātrakalanaiva jagat samagraṁ
saṁkalpamātrakalanaiva manovilāsaḥ |
saṁkalpamātramatimutsṛja nirvikalpam
āśritya niścayamavāpnuhi rāma śāntim ||58||

IV.58: The entire world is the fabrication of thoughts only. The function of the mind is also created only by thoughts. Transcending the mind, find rest in the changeless. O Rāma, then you can attain peace.

कर्पूरमनले यद्वत् सैन्धवं सलिले यथा ।
तथा संधीयमानं च मनस्तत्त्वे विलीयते ॥५९॥

karpūramanale yadvat saindhavaṁ salile yathā |
tathā saṁdhīyamānaṁ ca manastattve vilīyate ||59||

IV.59: Like camphor in fire and like salt in water, the mind dissolves in the true state through meditation (samādhi).

ज्ञेयं सर्वं प्रतीतं च ज्ञानं च मन उच्यते ।
ज्ञानं ज्ञेयं समं नष्टं नान्यः पन्था द्वितीयकः ॥६०॥

jñeyaṁ sarvaṁ pratītaṁ ca jñānaṁ ca mana ucyate |
jñānaṁ jñeyaṁ samaṁ naṣṭaṁ nānyaḥ panthā dvitīyakaḥ ||60||

IV.60: All that can be known, all that is known, and knowledge itself is said to be the mind. Knowledge and the known are destroyed together; there is no other way.

मनोदृश्यमिदं सर्वं यत्किंचित् सचराचरम् ।
मनसो ह्युन्मनीभावाद् द्वैतं नैवोपलभ्यते ॥६१॥

manodṛśyamidaṁ sarvaṁ yatkiṁcit sacarācaram |
manaso hyunmanībhāvād dvaitaṁ naivopalabhyate ||61||

IV.61: Whatever is perceived in this world, whether moving or still, appears in the mind. When the mind reaches the transcendent state (unmanī) then duality is not experienced.

ज्ञेयवस्तुपरित्यागाद् विलयं याति मानसम् ।
मनसो विलये जाते कैवल्यमवशिष्यते ॥६२॥

jñeyavastuparityāgād vilayaṁ yāti mānasam |
manaso vilaye jāte kaivalyamavaśiṣyate ||62||

IV.62: When all objects of knowledge are abandoned, the mind is absorbed [into stillness]. When the mind is thus dissolved, then the state of liberation (kaivalya) remains.

एवं नानाविधोपायाः सम्यक् स्वानुभवान्विताः ।
समाधिमार्गाः कथिताः पूर्वाचार्यैर्महात्मभिः ॥६३॥

evaṁ nānāvidhopāyāḥ samyak svānubhavānvitāḥ |
samādhimārgāḥ kathitāḥ pūrvācāryairmahātmabhiḥ ||63||

IV.63: Different means of reaching absorption (samādhi), have been described by the great ancient teachers, based on their own experience.

सुषुम्नायै कुण्डलिन्यै सुधायै चन्द्रजन्मने ।
मनोन्मन्यै नमस्तुभ्यं महाशक्त्यै चिदात्मने ॥६४॥

suṣumnāyai kuṇḍalinyai sudhāyai candrajanmane |
manonmanyai namastubhyaṁ mahāśaktyai cidātmane ||64||

IV.64: Salutations to suṣumnā, to kuṇḍalinī, to the nectar flowing from the moon, to manonmanī, and to the great power of pure consciousness.

[Krishnamacharya] This section concludes with a prayer to kuṇḍalinī and the key elements of the topics so far. The section on experiencing inner sound or vibration (nādopāsanā) now commences.

अशक्यतत्त्वबोधानां मूढानामपि संमतम् ।
प्रोक्तं गोरक्षनाथेन नादोपासनमुच्यते ॥६५॥

aśakyatattvabodhānāṁ mūḍhānāmapi saṁmatam |
proktaṁ gorakṣanāthena nādopāsanamucyate ||65||

IV.65: Now begins the explanation of the practice of experiencing the inner sound (nādopāsanā) that has been taught by Gorakṣanātha. It is suitable even for the unlearned who are unable to comprehend the subtle truths (tattva-s).

श्रीआदिनाथेन सपादकोटिलयप्रकाराः कथिता जयन्ति ।
नादानुसंधानकमेकमेव मन्यामहे मुख्यतमं लयानाम् ॥६६॥

śrīāadināthena sapādakoṭilayaprakārāḥ kathitā jayanti |
nādānusaṁdhānakamekameva manyāmahe mukhyatamaṁ layānām ||66||

IV.66: Śrī Ādinātha has expounded one and a quarter crores of effective types of absorption (laya). But we consider nādopāsanā the most important way of absorption.

मुक्तासने स्थितो योगी मुद्रां संधाय शांभवीम् ।
श्रृणुयाद् दक्षिणे कर्णे नादमन्तस्थमेकधीः ॥६७॥

muktāsane sthito yogī mudrāṁ saṁdhāya śāṁbhavīm |
śṛṇuyād dakṣiṇe karṇe nādamantasthamekadhīḥ ||67||

IV.67: Seated in muktāsana and assuming the śāṁbhavī-mudrā, the yogi should listen with a concentrated mind to the sound within (nāda), in the right ear.

श्रवणपुटनयनयुगलघ्राणमुखानां निरोधनं कार्यम् ।
शुद्धसुषुम्नासरणौ स्फुटममलः श्रूयते नादः ॥६८॥

śravaṇapuṭanayanayugalaghrāṇamukhānāṁ nirodhanaṁ kāryam |
śuddhasuṣumnāsaraṇau sphuṭamamalaḥ śrūyate nādaḥ ||68||

IV.68: Close the ears, eyes, nose, and the mouth. Then a clear and untainted sound (nāda) is heard in the pure path of suṣumnā.

[Krishnamacharya] In śāṁbhavī mudrā, the position of the head is neutral, neither raised nor lowered.

आरम्भश्च घटश्चैव तथा परिचयोऽपि च ।
निष्पत्तिः सर्वयोगेषु स्यादवस्थाचतुष्टयम् ॥६९॥

ārambhaśca ghaṭaścaiva tathā paricayo'pi ca |
niṣpattiḥ sarvayogeṣu syādavasthācatuṣṭayam ||69||

IV.69: There are four stages (avasthā-s) in all the paths: ārambha, ghaṭa, paricaya, and niṣpatti.

[Krishnamacharya] The four stages for absorption in laya yoga are described in the subsequent verses. In the mantra yoga, the equivalent stages are:

1. ārambha-avasthā: initiation into the mantra
2. ghaṭa-avasthā: practice with the mantra
3. paricaya-avasthā: rituals based on the mantra
4. niṣpatti-avasthā: complete absorption (samādhi) by meditation on the mantra

अथ आरम्भावस्था ।
ब्रह्मग्रन्थेर्भवेद्भेदो ह्यानन्दः शून्यसंभवः ।
विचित्रः क्वणको देहेऽनाहतः श्रूयते ध्वनिः ॥७०॥

atha ārambhāvasthā |
brahmagrantherbhavedbhedo hyānandaḥ śūnyasaṁbhavaḥ |
vicitraḥ kvaṇako dehe'nāhataḥ śrūyate dhvaniḥ ||70||

Now ārambha-āvasthā (stage 1) [is described]:

IV.70: When the knot of Brahma (anāhata-cakra) is pierced, bliss arises. Various tinkling sounds and the sound from the heart will be heard.

[Krishnamacharya] The Muṇḍaka Upaniṣat notes that piercing or drawing awareness into the heart is important to transcend desire, fear, and hatred.

दिव्यदेहश्च तेजस्वी दिव्यगन्धस्त्वरोगवान् ।
संपूर्णहृदयः शून्य आरम्भे योगवान् भवेत् ॥७१॥

divyadehaśca tejasvī divyagandhastvarogavān |
saṁpūrṇahṛdayaḥ śūnya ārambhe yogavān bhavet ||71||

IV.71: When this sound (nāda) begins to be heard in the void (śūnya), the yogi's body becomes lustrous and radiant, with an exquisite fragrance, free of diseases, and [the yogi experiences] a feeling of fulfilment.

[Krishnamacharya] This verse describes the result of the first stage.

अथ घटावस्था ।
द्वितीयायां घटीकृत्य वायुर्भवति मध्यगः ।
दृढासनो भवेद् योगी ज्ञानी देवसमस्तदा ॥७२॥

atha ghaṭāvasthā |

dvitīyāyāṁ ghaṭīkṛtya vāyurbhavati madhyagaḥ |
dṛḍhāsano bhaved yogī jñānī devasamastadā ||72||

Now ghaṭa-avasthā (stage 2) [is described]:

IV.72: In the second stage, the prāṇa is united in suṣumnā. The yogi then attains steadiness in posture, becomes wise, and is comparable to the gods.

विष्णुग्रन्थेस्ततो भेदात् परमानन्दसूचकः ।
अतिशून्ये विमर्दश्च भेरीशब्दस्तदा भवेत् ॥७३॥

viṣṇugranthestato bhedāt paramānandasūcakaḥ |
atiśūnye vimardaśca bherīśabdastadā bhavet ||73||

IV.73: When the knot of Viṣṇu (viśuddhi-cakra) is pierced, there arises supreme bliss. From the great void (atiśūnya), emerges a rumbling sound like a kettle drum.

[Krishnamacharya] When this prāṇāyāma is practiced, the body has a tendency to lift up from the support of the ground; this tendency must be controlled.

तृतीयायां तु विज्ञेयो विहायो मर्दलध्वनिः ।
महाशून्यं तदा याति सर्वसिद्धिसमाश्रयम् ॥७४ ॥

tṛtīyāyāṁ tu vijñeyo vihāyo mardaladhvaniḥ |
mahāśūnyaṁ tadā yāti sarvasiddhisamāśrayam ||74 ||

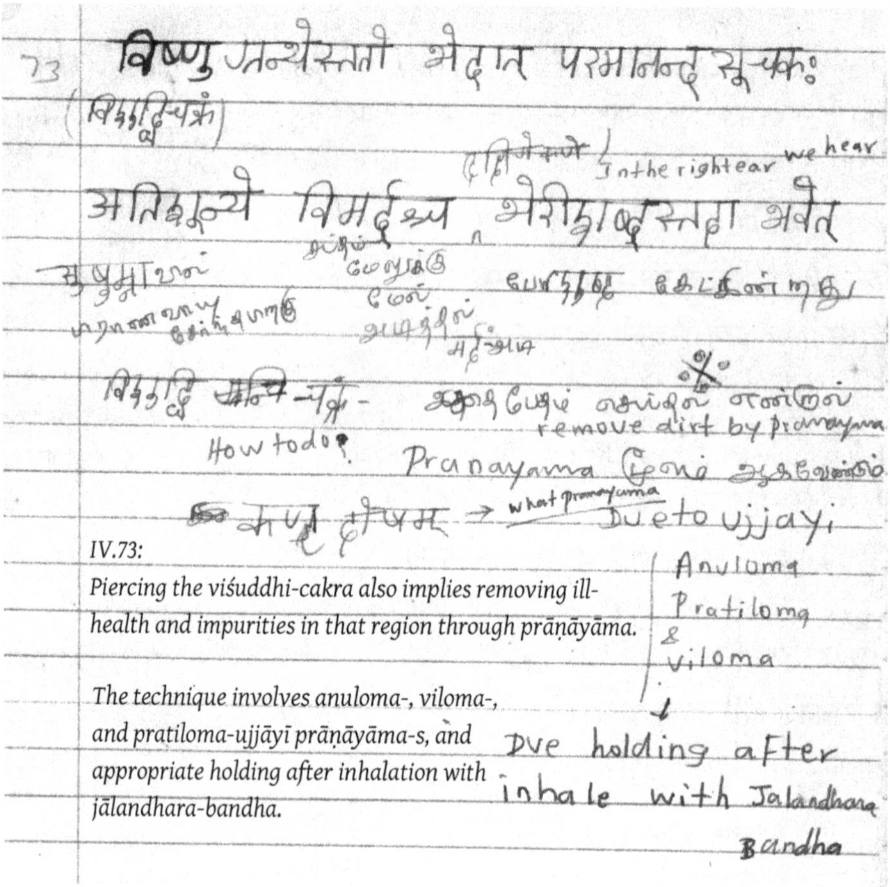

IV.73:
Piercing the viśuddhi-cakra also implies removing ill-health and impurities in that region through prāṇāyāma.

The technique involves anuloma-, viloma-, and pratiloma-ujjāyī prāṇāyāma-s, and appropriate holding after inhalation with jālandhara-bandha.

IV.74: [Paricaya-avasthā:] In the third stage, a sound like that of a drum is heard, where the [prāṇa] reaches the greatest void (ājñā-cakra), which is the seat of all the special powers (siddhi-s).

चित्तानन्दं तदा जित्वा सहजानन्दसंभवः ।
दोषदुःखजराव्याधिक्षुधानिद्राविवर्जितः ॥७५॥

cittānandaṁ tadā jitvā sahajānandasaṁbhavaḥ |
doṣaduḥkhajarāvyādhikṣudhānidrāvivarjitaḥ ||75||

IV.75: Having gone beyond the blissful state of mind [arising from the hearing the various sounds], experience of the natural state of bliss arises. Then the yogi becomes free from disorders of the doṣa-s, suffering, ageing, disease, hunger, and sleep.

परिचया वस्था

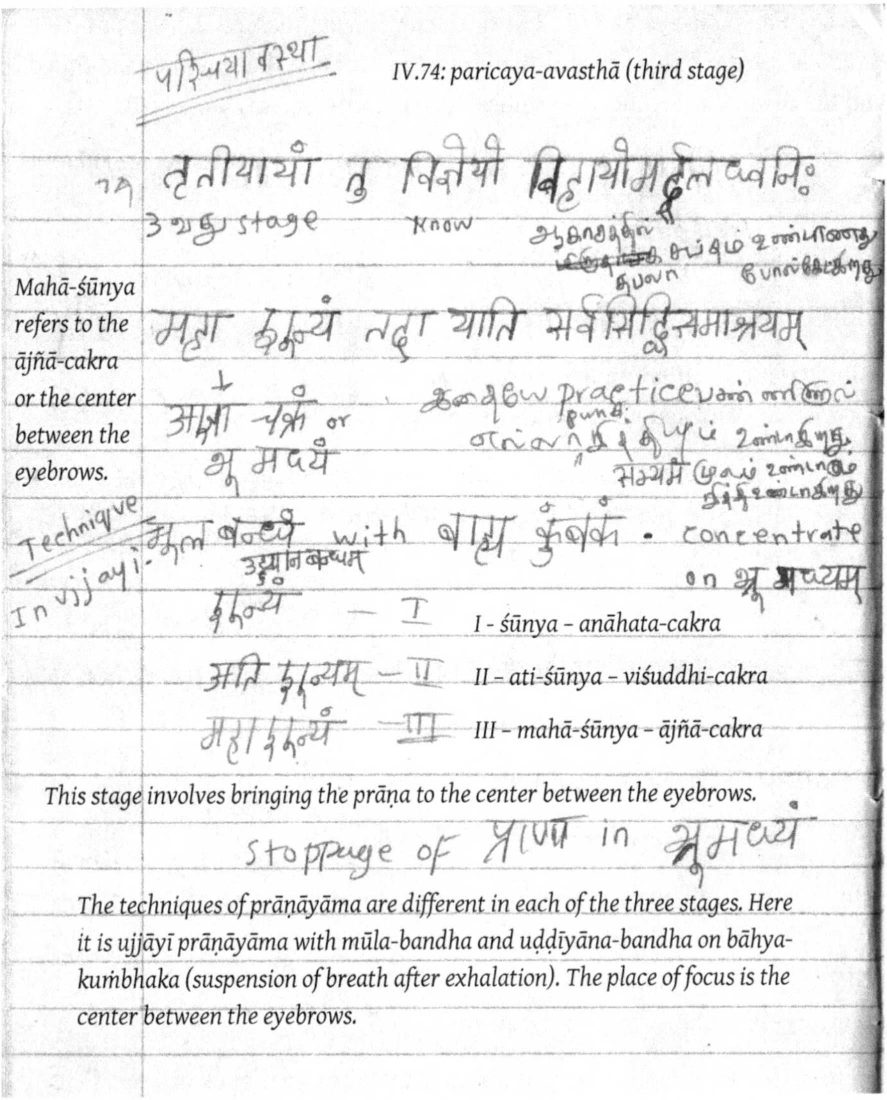

IV.74: paricaya-avasthā (third stage)

तृतीयायाँ तु विनियो विहायोमण्डल वनि‌

3rd stage   know

Mahā-śūnya refers to the ājñā-cakra or the center between the eyebrows.

महा शून्यं तथा याति सर्वसिद्धिसमाश्रयम्

अज्ञा चक्र or भू मध्यं

Technique – Ujjayi

मूल बन्ध with वाम भन्ध – concentrate
उ्यान्‌बन्धम्‌   on भू मध्यम्‌

शून्यं – I   I - śūnya - anāhata-cakra

अति शून्यम् – II   II – ati-śūnya - viśuddhi-cakra

महा शून्यं – III   III – mahā-śūnya - ājñā-cakra

This stage involves bringing the prāṇa to the center between the eyebrows.

Stoppage of प्राण in भूमध्यं

The techniques of prāṇāyāma are different in each of the three stages. Here it is ujjāyī prāṇāyāma with mūla-bandha and uḍḍīyāna-bandha on bāhya-kumbhaka (suspension of breath after exhalation). The place of focus is the center between the eyebrows.

[Krishnamacharya] This verse describes the result of the third stage.

रुद्रग्रन्थिं यदा भित्त्वा शर्वपीठगतोऽनिलः ।
निष्पत्तौ वैणवः शब्दः क्वणद्वीणाक्वणो भवेत् ॥७६॥

rudragranthiṁ yadā bhittvā śarvapīṭhagato'nilaḥ |
niṣpattau vainavaḥ śabdaḥ kvaṇadvīṇākvaṇo bhavet ||76||

IV.76: In niṣpatti-avasthā (i.e fourth stage), having pierced the knot of Rudra (ājñā-cakra) the prāṇa reaches the seat of Śiva. Then the sound of the flute and the resonance of the vīṇā (musical string instrument) are heard.

[Krishnamacharya] The usage of the word seat (pīṭha) here implies being stationary, whereas a cakra implies movement.

एकीभूतं तदा चित्तं राजयोगाभिधानकम् ।
सृष्टिसंहारकर्तासौ योगीश्वरसमो भवेत् ॥७७॥

ekībhūtaṁ tadā cittaṁ rājayogābhidhānakam |
sṛṣṭisaṁhārakartāsau yogīśvarasamo bhavet ||77||

IV.77: The mind becoming one [with the ātman] is called rāja-yoga. Then the yogi, attaining the power of creation and destruction, becomes equal to the Divine (īśvara).

[Krishnamacharya] This is rāja-yoga according to the Haṭha Yoga Pradīpikā.

अस्तु वा मास्तु वा मुक्तिरत्रैवाखण्डितं सुखम् ।
लयोद्भवमिदं सौख्यं राजयोगादवाप्यते ॥७८॥
राजयोगमजानन्तः केवलं हठकर्मिणः ।
एतानभ्यासिनो मन्ये प्रयासफलवर्जितान् ॥७९॥

astu vā māstu vā muktiratraivākhaṇḍitaṁ sukham |
layodbhavamidaṁ saukhyaṁ rājayogādavāpyate ||78||
rājayogamajānantaḥ kevalaṁ haṭhakarmiṇaḥ |
etānabhyāsino manye prayāsaphalavarjitān ||79||

IV.78: Whether there is liberation or not, there is experience of boundless bliss in this state. This bliss arising from absorption (laya) is attained through rāja-yoga.

IV.79: There are those who merely practice haṭha-yoga without the knowledge of rāja-yoga. I regard them to be practitioners who do not attain the fruit of their efforts.

उन्मन्यवाप्तये शीघ्रं भ्रूध्यानं मम संमतम् ।
राजयोगपदं प्राप्तुं सुखोपायोऽल्पचेतसाम् ।

सद्यः प्रत्ययसंधायी जायते नादजो लयः ॥८०॥

unmanvavāptaye śīghraṁ bhrūdhyānaṁ mama saṁmatam |
rājayogapadaṁ prāptuṁ sukhopāyo'lpacetasām |
sadyaḥ pratyayasaṁdhāyī jāyate nādajo layaḥ ||80||

IV.80: In order to attain absorption (samādhi) in a short time, one must concentrate on the cakra between the eyebrows. Even for the unlearned, this is an easy way for attaining the state of rāja-yoga. The absorption (laya) arising from the inner sound (nāda) gives immediate experience.

नादानुसंधानसमाधिभाजां योगीश्वराणां हृदि वर्धमानम् ।
आनन्दमेकं वचसामगम्यं जानाति तं श्रीगुरुनाथ एकः ॥८१ ॥

nādānusaṁdhānasamādhibhājāṁ yogīśvarāṇāṁ hṛdi vardhamānam |
ānandamekaṁ vacasāmagamyaṁ jānāti taṁ śrīgurunātha ekaḥ ||81||

IV.81: In the heart of the great yogi-s who remain in absorption (samādhi) through the experience of the inner sound (nādānusandhāna), there is unequalled bliss, beyond description, attained through the grace of the guru.

कर्णौ पिधाय हस्ताभ्यां यं श्रृणोति ध्वनिं मुनिः ।
तत्र चित्तं स्थिरीकुर्याद् यावत् स्थिरपदं व्रजेत् ॥८२॥

karṇau pidhāya hastābhyāṁ yaṁ śrṛṇoti dhvaniṁ muniḥ |
tatra cittaṁ sthirīkuryād yāvat sthirapadaṁ vrajet ||82||

IV.82: The yogi in silence (muni), closing his ears with the thumbs, should focus his mind on the sound within until he attains stability [of the mind].

अभ्यस्यमानो नादोऽयं बाह्यमावृणुते ध्वनिम् ।
पक्षाद् विक्षेपमखिलं जित्वा योगी सुखी भवेत् ॥८३॥

abhyasyamāno nādo'yaṁ bāhyamāvṛṇute dhvanim |
pakṣād vikṣepamakhilaṁ jitvā yogī sukhī bhavet ||83||

IV.83: Through the sustained practice of listening to the inner sound, the external sounds are drowned by the inner sound. In fifteen days, the yogi overcomes all distractions and becomes happy.

[Krishnamacharya] Now follows a section on how to practice experiencing the inner sound (nādānusandhāna) from gross to subtle.

श्रूयते प्रथमाभ्यासे नादो नानाविधो महान् ।
ततोऽभ्यासे वर्धमाने श्रूयते सूक्ष्मसूक्ष्मकः ॥८४॥

śrūyate prathamābhyāse nādo nānāvidho mahān |
tato'bhyāse vardhamāne śrūyate sūkṣmasūkṣmakaḥ ||84||

IV.84: During the initial stages of practice, various louder inner sounds are heard. Then with increasing practice, progressively [more] subtle sounds are heard.

आदौ जलधिजीमूतभेरीझर्झरसंभवाः ।
मध्ये मर्दलशङ्खोत्था घण्टाकाहलजास्तथा ॥८५॥
अन्ते तु किंकिणीवंशवीणाभ्रमरनिःस्वनाः ।
इति नानाविधा नादाः श्रूयन्ते देहमध्यगाः ॥८६॥

ādau jaladhijīmūtabherījharjharasaṁbhavāḥ |
madhye mardalaśaṅkhotthā ghaṇṭākāhalajāstathā ||85||

ante tu kiṁkiṇīvaṁśavīṇābhramaraniḥsvanāḥ |
iti nānāvidhā nādāḥ śrūyante dehamadhyagāḥ ||86||

IV.85-86: In the beginning, various sounds resembling those of the ocean, thunder, the kettle drum, and the jharjhara drum are heard. In the middle stage [the sounds] of the drum, the conch, the bell, and the horn are heard. Finally, the sounds like tingling bells, the flute, the vīṇā, and bees are heard within the body.

[Krishnamacharya] Śvetāśvatara Upaniṣat describes different colours for meditation. Basically, by the practice of nādānusandhāna, deep and steady mental focus (ekāgratā) arises.

महति श्रूयमाणेऽपि मेघभेर्यादिके ध्वनौ ।
तत्र सूक्ष्मात् सूक्ष्मतरं नादमेव परामृशेत् ॥८७॥

mahati śrūyamāṇe'pi meghabheryādike dhvanau |
tatra sūkṣmāt sūkṣmataraṁ nādameva parāmṛśet ||87||

IV.87: Although loud sounds like thunder and the kettle drum are heard, attention should be turned to the subtle and still subtler sounds.

घनमुत्सृज्य वा सूक्ष्मे सूक्ष्ममुत्सृज्य वा घने ।
रममाणमपि क्षिप्तं मनो नान्यत्र चालयेत् ॥८८॥

ghanamutsṛjya vā sūkṣme sūkṣmamutsṛjya vā ghane |
ramamāṇamapi kṣiptaṁ mano nānyatra cālayet ||88||

IV.88: Attention may shift from the gross to the subtle sounds, or from the subtle to the gross sounds [arising from within], but it should not be allowed to wander elsewhere.

[Krishnamacharya] To succeed in these practices, strict control over one's diet is necessary.

यत्रकुत्रापि वा नादे लगति प्रथमं मनः ।
तत्रैव सुस्थिरीभूय तेन सार्धं विलीयते ॥८९॥

yatrakutrāpi vā nāde lagati prathamaṁ manaḥ |
tatraiva susthirībhūya tena sārdhaṁ vilīyate ||89||

IV.89: On whichever inner sound the mind focuses, in that it attains steadiness, and in it [the mind] is absorbed.

[Krishnamacharya] Verses 90-99 contain various metaphors. Verses 103-115 are largely repetition and praise.

मकरन्दं पिबन् भृङ्गो गन्धं नापेक्षते यथा ।
नादासक्तं तथा चित्तं विषयान् नहि काङ्क्षते ॥९०॥

makarandaṁ piban bhṛṅgo gandhaṁ nāpekṣate yathā |
nādāsaktaṁ tathā cittaṁ viṣayān nahi kāṅkṣate ||90||

IV.90: Just as a bee drinking honey does not care for the [flower's] fragrance, so also the mind absorbed in the inner sound does not crave objects [of enjoyment].

मनोमत्तगजेन्द्रस्य विषयोद्यानचारिणः ।
समर्थोऽयं नियमने निनादनिशिताङ्कुशः ॥९१॥

manomattagajendrasya viṣayodyānacāriṇaḥ |
samartho'yaṁ niyamane ninādaniśitāṅkuśaḥ ||91 ||

IV.91: The sharp elephant-goad of inner sound effectively controls the mind which is like an elephant in rut wandering in the garden of sense objects.

बद्धं तु नादबन्धेन मनः संत्यक्तचापलम् ।
प्रयाति सुतरां स्थैर्यं छिन्नपक्षः खगो यथा ॥९२॥

baddhaṁ tu nādabandhena manaḥ saṁtyaktacāpalam |
prayāti sutarāṁ sthairyaṁ chinnapakṣaḥ khago yathā ||92 ||

IV.92: When the mind is held by the inner sound, it overcomes its restlessness and becomes steady, like a bird that has shed its wings.

सर्वचिन्तां परित्यज्य सावधानेन चेतसा ।
नाद एवानुसंधेयो योगसाम्राज्यमिच्छता ॥९३॥

sarvacintāṁ parityajya sāvadhānena cetasā |
nāda evānusaṁdheyo yogasāmrājyamicchatā ||93||

IV.93: One who desires to obtain sovereignty in yoga should put away all mental concerns and, with full concentration, meditate on the inner sound.

नादोऽन्तरङ्गसारङ्गबन्धने वागुरायते ।
अन्तरङ्गकुरङ्गस्य वधे व्याधायतेऽपि च ॥९४॥

nādo'ntaraṅgasāraṅgabandhane vāgurāyate |
antaraṅgakuraṅgasya vadhe vyādhāyate'pi ca ||94||

IV.94: The inner sound is like the net which ensnares the deer within (i.e. the mind) and it is also the hunter who slays the deer within.

अन्तरङ्गस्य यमिनो वाजिनः परिघायते ।
नादोपास्तिरतो नित्यमवधार्या हि योगिना ॥९५॥

antaraṅgasya yamino vājinaḥ parighāyate |
nādopāstirato nityamavadhāryā hi yoginā ||95||

IV.95: The inner sound is like the bolt which locks the horse (i.e. the mind) within the yogi. A yogi should, therefore, meditate on the inner sound every day.

बद्धं विमुक्तचाञ्चल्यं नादगन्धकजारणात् ।
मनःपारदमाप्नोति निरालम्बाख्यखेऽटनम् ॥९६॥

baddhaṁ vimuktacāñcalyaṁ nādagandhakajāraṇāt |
manaḥpāradamāpnoti nirālambākhyakhe'ṭanam ||96||

IV.96: The mind is like mercury, which is bound (i.e. solidified) by the action of the inner sound which is like sulphur. It is freed from its restlessness and able to move without support in space (Brahman).

नादश्रवणतः क्षिप्रमन्तरङ्गभुजङ्गमः ।
विस्मृत्य सर्वमेकाग्रः कुत्रचिन्नहि धावति ॥९७॥

nādaśravaṇataḥ kṣipramantaraṅgabhujaṅgamaḥ |
vismṛtya sarvamekāgraḥ kutracinnahi dhāvati ||97||

IV.97: The mind like a serpent within, on hearing the inner sound, becomes oblivious of all else, gets completely focused, and does not move anywhere else.

काष्ठे प्रवर्तितो वह्निः काष्ठेन सह शाम्यति ।
नादे प्रवर्तितं चित्तं नादेन सह लीयते ॥९८॥

kāṣṭhe pravartito vahniḥ kāṣṭhena saha śāmyati |
nāde pravartitaṁ cittaṁ nādena saha līyate ||98||

IV.98: The fire in a piece of wood subsides along with the [burnt out] wood. Similarly, the mind focused on the inner sound is absorbed along with it.

घण्टादिनादसक्तस्तब्धान्तः करणहरिणस्य ।
प्रहरणमपि सुकरं स्याच्छरसंधानप्रवीणश्चेत् ॥९९ ॥

ghaṇṭādinādasaktastabdhāntaḥ karaṇahariṇasya |
praharaṇamapi sukaraṁ syāccharasaṁdhānapravīṇaścet ||99 ||

IV.99: The mind is like a deer held still by the sound of bells, and hence slain easily by one who is expert in aiming and shooting the arrow.

अनाहतस्य शब्दस्य ध्वनिर्य उपलभ्यते ।
ध्वनेरन्तर्गतं ज्ञेयं ज्ञेयस्यान्तर्गतं मनः ।
मनस्तत्र लयं याति तद्विष्णोः परमं पदम् ॥१००॥

anāhatasya śabdasya dhvanirya upalabhyate |
dhvanerantargataṁ jñeyaṁ jñeyasyāntargataṁ manaḥ |
manastatra layaṁ yāti tadviṣṇoḥ paramaṁ padam ||100||

IV.100: The experience of the unstruck (i.e. innately occurring) sound that is heard—the quintessence of that sound is the object of knowing and the mind is within the object of knowing. The mind dissolves in it (the object of knowing). That is the supreme state of Viṣṇu (the all-pervading).

तावदाकाशसङ्कल्पो यावच्छब्दः प्रवर्तते ।
निःशब्दं तत्परं ब्रह्म परमात्मेति गीयते ॥१०१॥

tāvadākāśasaṅkalpo yāvacchabdaḥ pravartate |
niḥśabdaṁ tatparaṁ brahma paramātmeti gīyate ||101||

IV.101: The concept of space exists as long as sound is heard. The soundless which is the supreme reality is called Brahman.

यत्किञ्चिन्नादरूपेण श्रूयते शक्तिरेव सा ।
यस्तत्त्वान्तो निराकारः स एव परमेश्वरः ॥१०२॥
इति नादानुसंधानम्

yatkiñcinnādarūpeṇa śrūyate śaktireva sā |
yastattvānto nirākāraḥ sa eva parameśvaraḥ ||102||
iti nādānusaṁdhānam

IV.102: What is heard as the inner sound is indeed energy (śakti). That in which all the elements (tattva-s) dissolve is the formless entity, the ultimate (parameśvara).

Thus ends the [section on] meditation on the inner sound.

सर्वे हठलयोपाया राजयोगस्य सिद्धये ।
राजयोगसमारूढः पुरुषः कालवञ्चकः ॥१०३॥

sarve haṭhalayopāyā rājayogasya siddhaye |
rājayogasamārūḍhaḥ puruṣaḥ kālavañcakaḥ ||103||

IV.103: All the practices of haṭha-yoga and laya-yoga are only for the attainment of rāja-yoga. One who has attained rāja-yoga conquers time.

तत्त्वं बीजं हठः क्षेत्रमौदासीन्यं जलं त्रिभिः ।
उन्मनी कल्पलतिका सद्य एव प्रवर्तते ॥१०४॥

tattvaṁ bījaṁ haṭhaḥ kṣetramaudāsīnyaṁ jalaṁ tribhiḥ |
unmanī kalpalatikā sadya eva pravartate ||104||

IV.104: The mind is the seed, haṭha-yoga is the soil, and equanimity is the water. With these three, absorption (unmanī), the tree that grants all wishes (kalpa-vṛkṣa), arises immediately.

सदा नादानुसंधानात् क्षीयन्ते पापसंचयाः ।
निरञ्जने विलीयेते निश्चितं चित्तमारुतौ ॥१०५॥

sadā nādānusaṁdhānāt kṣīyante pāpasaṁcayāḥ |
nirañjane vilīyete niścitaṁ cittamārutau ||105||

IV.105: Through constant meditation on nāda, all accumulated sins (pāpa) are destroyed. The mind and the prāṇa are absorbed in that [ātman or self] which is unsullied.

शङ्खदुन्दुभिनादं च न श्रृणोति कदाचन ।
काष्ठवज्जायते देह उन्मन्यावस्थया ध्रुवम् ॥१०६॥

śaṅkhadundubhinādaṁ ca na śṛṇoti kadācana |
kāṣṭhavajjāyate deha unmanyāvasthayā dhruvam ||106||

IV.106: In the state of absorption (unmanī), the body is like a log of wood and the yogi does not hear even the sounds of a conch or drum.

सर्वावस्थाविनिर्मुक्तः सर्वचिन्ताविवर्जितः ।
मृतवत् तिष्ठते योगी स मुक्तो नात्र संशयः ॥१०७॥

sarvāvasthāvinirmuktaḥ sarvacintāvivarjitaḥ |
mṛtavat tiṣṭhate yogī sa mukto nātra saṁśayaḥ ||107||

IV.107: The yogi who is beyond all states, free from all thoughts, and who is still as if dead, is no doubt liberated.

खाद्यते न च कालेन बाध्यते न च कर्मणा ।
साध्यते न स केनापि योगी युक्तः समाधिना ॥१०८॥

khādyate na ca kālena bādhyate na ca karmaṇā |
sādhyate na sa kenāpi yogī yuktaḥ samādhinā ||108||

IV.108: A yogi in absorption (samādhi) is not affected by time. He is not affected by [the fruits of his] actions. He does not fall under any influence [from persons, incantations etc.].

न गन्धं न रसं रूपं न च स्पर्शं न निःस्वनम् ।
नात्मानं न परं वेत्ति योगी युक्तः समाधिना ॥१०९॥

na gandhaṁ na rasaṁ rūpaṁ na ca sparśaṁ na niḥsvanam |
nātmānaṁ na paraṁ vetti yogī yuktaḥ samādhinā ||109||

IV.109: A yogi in absorption (samādhi) does not cognize smell, taste, form, touch, sound, himself, or others.

चित्तं न सुप्तं नोजाग्रत्स्मृतिविस्मृतिवर्जितम् ।
न चास्तमेति नोदेति यस्यासौ मुक्त एव सः ॥११०॥

cittaṁ na suptaṁ nojāgratsmṛtivismṛtivarjitam |
na cāstameti nodeti yasyāsau mukta eva saḥ ||110||

IV.110: One whose mind is neither asleep nor awake, [whose mind] is free of memories and of forgetfulness, [whose mind] neither goes into oblivion nor is lost in activity, is indeed liberated.

न विजानाति शीतोष्णं न दुःखं न सुखं तथा ।
न मानं नापमानं च योगी युक्तः समाधिना ॥ १११ ॥

na vijānāti śītoṣṇaṁ na duḥkhaṁ na sukhaṁ tathā |
na mānaṁ nāpamānaṁ ca yogī yuktaḥ samādhinā ||111||

IV.111: A yogi in absorption (samādhi) is not affected by heat or cold, pain or pleasure, honour or dishonour.

स्वस्थो जाग्रदवस्थायां सुप्तवद्योऽवतिष्ठते ।
निःश्वासोच्छ्वासहीनश्च निश्चितं मुक्त एव सः ॥ ११२ ॥

svastho jāgradavasthāyāṁ suptavadyo'vatiṣṭhate |
niḥśvāsocchvāsahīnaśca niścitaṁ mukta eva saḥ ||112||

IV.112: One who is healthy [with mind and senses being clear], who, in the waking state, appears to be asleep, not inhaling or exhaling [due to spontaneous stillness of, or minimal breathing,] is indeed liberated.

अवध्यः सर्वशस्त्राणामशक्यः सर्वदेहिनाम् ।
अग्राह्यो मन्त्रयन्त्राणां योगी युक्तः समाधिना ॥ ११३ ॥

avadhyaḥ sarvaśastrāṇāmaśakyaḥ sarvadehinām |
agrāhyo mantrayantrāṇāṁ yogī yuktaḥ samādhinā ||113||

IV.II3: A yogi in absorption (samādhi) is not vulnerable to any weapons, cannot be assailed by other beings, and is not susceptible to mantra-s and yantra-s.

यावन्नैव प्रविशति चरन्मारुतो मध्यमार्गे
यावद् बिन्दुर्न भवति दृढः प्राणवातप्रबन्धात् ।
यावद् ध्याने सहजसदृशं जायते नैव तत्त्वं
तावज्ज्ञानं वदति तदिदं दम्भमिथ्याप्रलापः ॥ ११४ ॥

yāvannaiva praviśati caranmāruto madhyamārge
yāvad bindurna bhavati dṛḍhaḥ prāṇavātaprabandhāt |
yāvad dhyāne sahajasadṛśaṁ jāyate naiva tattvaṁ
tāvajjñānaṁ vadati tadidaṁ dambhamithyāpralāpaḥ ||114 ||

IV.114: As long as the prāṇa does not flow in the central path (suṣumnā), as long as the vitality does not become steady through the restraint of breath, as long as the mind does not remain in the natural state of meditation, those who talk of spiritual knowledge indulge only in boastful and false prattle.